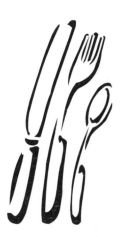

10 9 8 7 6 5 4 3 2 1

Published In 1999 by Sterling Publishing Company, Inc.
387 Park Avenue South, New York, N.Y. 10016

Material in this collection was adapted from
The Complete Diabetic Cookbook
© Mary Jane Finsand
Diabetic High Fiber Cookbook
© Mary Jane Finsand
Diabetic Breakfast & Brunch Cookbook
© Mary Jane Finsand
Great Diabetic Desserts & Sweets
© Karin Cadwell, Ph.D., R.N.
and Edith White, M.Ed.
and
Diabetic Candy, Cookie & Dessert Cookbook
© Mary Jane Finsand

Distributed in Canada by Sterling Publishing
c/o Canadian Manda Group
One Atlantic Avenue, Suite 105
Toronto, Ontario, Canada M6K 3E7

Distributed in Great Britain and Europe by Cassell PLC
Wellington House, 125 Strand
London WC2R 0BB, United Kingdom

Distributed in Australia by Capricorn Link (Australia) Pty Ltd.
P.O. Box 6651, Baulkham Hills, Business Centre,
NSW 2153, Australia

Sterling ISBN 0-8069-7131-2

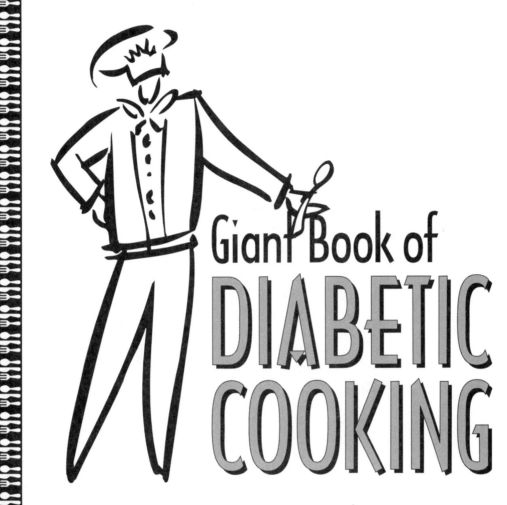

Giant Book of
DIABETIC
COOKING

Mary Jane Finsand,
Karin Cadwell, Ph.D., R.N.
& Edith White, M.Ed.

Main Street

CONTENTS

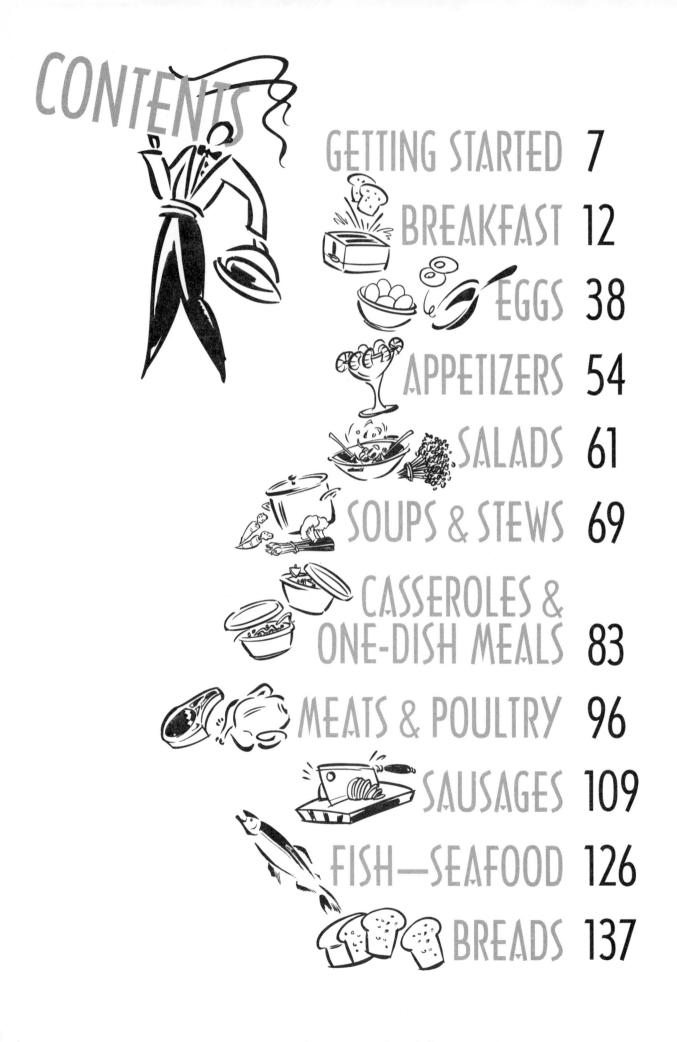

USING THE RECIPES FOR YOUR DIET

All recipes have been developed using diet substitutions for sugar, syrup, sauces, toppings, puddings, gelatins, mayonnaise, salad dressings, and imitation or lo-cal dairy and non-dairy products.

Remember, diet is the key word for controlling diabetes, and each person's diet is prescribed individually by a doctor or counselor who has been trained to mold your daily life to your diet requirements. DO NOT try to outguess them. If you have any questions about any diabetic recipes, ask your diet counselor.

Read the recipes carefully, then assemble all equipment and ingredients. "Added Touch" ingredients are flavorful additions, but not necessary to the recipe's success. Substitutions or additions of herbs and spices or flavorings to a recipe may be made by using the guide for Spices and Herbs, or for Flavorings and Extracts; they will make any of the recipes distinctively your own.

Use standard measuring equipment (whether metric or customary); be sure to measure accurately. Remember, these recipes are good for everyone, not just the diabetic.

CUSTOMARY TERMS	METRIC SYMBOLS
teaspoon	milliliter
tablespoon	liter
cup	gram
package	kilogram
pint	millimeter
quart	centimeter
ounce	degrees °Celsius
pound	
degrees °Fahrenheit	
inch	

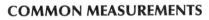

COMMON MEASUREMENTS

3 teaspoons = 1 Tablespoon
4 Tablespoons = 1/4 cup
5 1/3 Tablespoons = 1/3 cup
4 ounces = 1/2 cup
8 ounces = 1 cup
1 cup = 1/2 pint

GUIDE TO APPROXIMATE EQUIVALENTS

CUSTOMARY				METRIC	
ounces pounds	cups	tablespoons	teaspoons	milliliters	grams kilograms
			1/4 teaspoon	1 milliliter	
			1/2 teaspoon	2 milliliters	
			1 teaspoon	5 milliliters	
			2 teaspoons	10 milliliters	
1/2 ounce		1 tablespoon	3 teaspoons	15 milliliters	15 grams
1 ounce		2 tablespoons	6 teaspoons	30 milliliters	30 grams
2 ounces	1/4 cup	4 tablespoons	12 teaspoons	60 milliliters	
4 ounces	1/2 cup	8 tablespoons	24 teaspoons	125 milliliters	
8 ounces	1 cup	16 tablespoons	48 teaspoons	250 milliliters	
2.2 pounds					1 kilogram

Keep in mind that this is not an exact conversion, but generally may be used for food measurement.

OVEN COOKING GUIDES

Follow this guide for oven temperature:

°Fahrenheit	Oven Heat	°Celsius
250–275°	very slow	120–135°
300–325°	slow	150–165°
350–375°	moderate	175–190°
400–425°	hot	200–220°
450–475°	very hot	230–245°
475–500°	hottest	250–290°

Use this meat thermometer probe guide to check the meat's internal temperature:

°Fahrenheit	Desired Doneness	°Celsius
140°	***Beef:*** rare	60°
150°	medium	65°
170°	well done	75°
160°	***Lamb:*** medium	70°
170°	well done	75°
180°	***Veal:*** well done	80°
180°	***Pork:*** well done	80°
185°	***Poultry:*** well done	85°

GUIDE TO PAN SIZES

BAKING PANS

Customary:	Metric:	Holds:
8-inch pie	20-centimeter pie	600 milliliters
9-inch pie	23-centimeter pie	1 liter
10-inch pie	25-centimeter pie	1.3 liters
8-inch round	20-centimeter round	1 liter
9-inch round	23-centimeter round	1.5 liters
8-inch square	20-centimeter square	2 liters
9-inch square	23-centimeter square	2.5 liters
9 x 5 x 2-inch loaf	23 x 13 x 5-centimeter loaf	2 liters
9-inch tube	23-centimeter tube	3 liters
10-inch tube	25-centimeter tube	3 liters
13 x 9 x 2-inch	33 x 23 x 5-centimeter	3.5 liters
14 x 10-inch (cookie tin)	35 x 25-centimeter (cookie tin)	
15 x 10½ x 1-inch (jelly-roll)	39 x 25 x 3-centimeter (jelly-roll)	

COOKING PANS AND CASSEROLES

Customary:	Metric:
1 quart	1 liter
2 quart	2 liter
3 quart	3 liter

SPICES AND HERBS

Allspice: Cinnamon, ginger, nutmeg flavor; used in breads, pastries, jellies, jams, pickles.

Anise: Licorice flavor; used in candies, breads, fruit, wine, liqueurs.

Basil: Sweet-strong flavor; used in meat, cheese, egg, tomato dishes.

Bay Leaf: Sweet flavor; used in meat, fish, vegetable dishes.

Celery: Unique, pleasantly bitter flavor; used in anything not sweet.

Chive: Light onion flavor; used in anything where onion should be delicate.

Chili Powder: Hot, pungent flavor; used in Mexican, Spanish dishes.

Cinnamon: Pungent, sweet flavor; used in pastries, breads, pickles, wine, beer, liqueurs.

Clove: Pungent, sweet flavor; used for ham, sauces, pastries, puddings, fruit, wine, liqueurs.

Coriander: Butter-lemon flavor; used for pork, cookies, cakes, pies, puddings, fruit, wine and liqueur punches.

Garlic: Strong, aromatic flavor; used in Italian, French and many meat dishes.

Ginger: Strong, pungent flavor; used in anything sweet, plus with beer, brandy, liqueurs.

Marjoram: Sweet, semi-pungent flavor; used in poultry, lamb, egg, vegetable dishes.

Nutmeg: Sweet, nutty flavor; used in pastries, puddings, vegetables.

Oregano: Sweet, pungent flavor; used in meat, pasta, vegetable dishes.

Paprika: Light, sweet flavor; used in salads, vegetables, poultry, fish, egg dishes; often used to brighten bland-colored casseroles or entrees.

Rosemary: Fresh, sweet flavor; used in soups, meat and vegetable dishes.

Sage: Pungent, bitter flavor; used in stuffings, sausages, some cheese dishes.

Thyme: Pungent, semi-bitter flavor; used in salty dishes or soups.

Woodruff: Sweet vanilla flavor; used in wines, punches.

Note: Metric equivalents for the stronger spices and herbs vary for each recipe to allow for individual effectiveness at convenient measurements.

FLAVORINGS AND EXTRACTS

Orange, lime, and lemon peels give vegetables, pastries, and puddings a fresh, clean flavor; liquor flavors, such as brandy or rum, give cakes and other desserts a company flare. Choose from the following to add some zip without calories:

Almond	Butter Rum	Pecan
Anise (Licorice)	Cherry	Peppermint
Apricot	Clove	Pineapple
Banana Crème	Coconut	Raspberry
Blackberry	Grape	Rum
Black Walnut	Hazelnut	Sassafras
Blueberry	Lemon	Sherry
Brandy	Lime	Strawberry
Burnt Sugar	Mint	Vanilla
Butter	Orange	Walnut
Butternut		

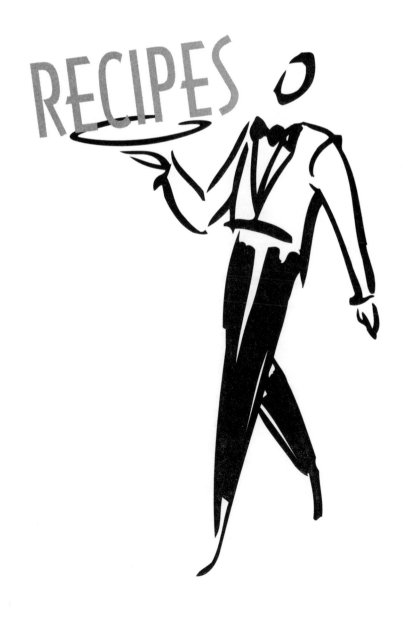

RECIPES

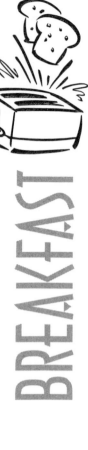

APRICOT MORNING DRINK

16-ounce can	Featherweight water pack apricot halves	454-gram can
1½ cups	skim milk	375 milliliters
3	eggs	3
1 teaspoon	vanilla extract	5 milliliters
½ teaspoon	Featherweight liquid sweetener	2 milliliters
	ground cinnamon	

Combine all ingredients except the cinnamon in a blender and cover. Blend at medium speed 30 seconds. Pour into glasses and sprinkle apricot drink with cinnamon.

Yield: 3 servings
Exchange: (1 serving) 1 fruit, 1 high-fat meat, ½ nonfat milk
Calories: (1 serving) 191

Based on a recipe from Featherweight Brand Foods.

MIXED FRUIT COCKTAIL

8-ounce can	Featherweight sliced peaches (drained); reserve 1 tablespoon (15 milliliters) liquid	227-gram can
8-ounce can	Featherweight pear halves (drained & cut in quarters)	227-gram can
8-ounce can	Featherweight sliced pineapple (drained & cut in quarters)	227-gram can
8-ounce can	Featherweight purple plums (drained, pitted & cut in halves)	227-gram can
½ cup	Featherweight apricot preserves	125 milliliters

Combine drained fruit in a bowl. Mix preserves and reserved peach liquid in a small saucepan; heat thoroughly. Pour over fruit and stir.

Yield: 4 servings
Exchange: (1 serving) 3 fruit
Calories: (1 serving) 117

Based on a recipe from Featherweight Brand Foods.

BROILED GRAPEFRUIT

1	grapefruit	1
1/2 teaspoon	butter	2 milliliters
1 teaspoon	granulated sugar replacement	5 milliliters
dash	ground cinnamon	dash
dash	ground or grated nutmeg	dash

A simple, but often forgotten breakfast starter. Cut grapefruit in half crosswise. Loosen sections with a sharp knife or grapefruit spoon. Place 1/4 teaspoon (1 milliliter) butter in middle of each half. Sprinkle each half with 1/2 teaspoon (2 milliliters) granulated sugar replacement, cinnamon and nutmeg. Broil 4 inches (10 centimeters) from heat for 6 to 8 minutes. Serve hot.

> **Yield:** 2 servings
> **Exchange:** (1 serving) 1 fruit, 1/2 fat
> **Calories:** (1 serving) 60

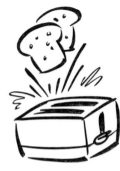

CITRUS CUP

4	oranges	4
1/2 cup	fresh shredded coconut (chopped)	125 milliliters
8-ounce can	Featherweight grapefruit segments (drained)	227-gram can
8-ounce can	Featherweight pineapple (drained & cut into eighths)	227-gram can

Cut off top third of oranges. Scoop out pulp, slice into pieces and put into a bowl. Set orange shells in custard cups. Reserve 1 tablespoon (15 milliliters) coconut. Add remaining coconut, grapefruit and pineapple to orange pieces; toss gently. Spoon fruit into orange shells. Top with reserved coconut.

> **Yield:** 4 servings
> **Exchange:** (1 serving) 4 fruit, 1/2 fat
> **Calories:** (1 serving) 192

Based on a recipe from Featherweight Brand Foods.

BREAKFAST

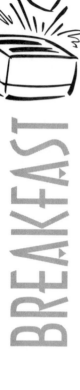

ITALIAN SCRAMBLED EGGS

1 small	butternut squash (thinly sliced)	1 small
1 small	onion (thinly sliced)	1 small
3 tablespoons	butter	45 milliliters
1 cup	meatless spaghetti sauce	250 milliliters
	(salt & pepper to taste)	
4	large eggs	4
2 tablespoons	water	30 milliliters

In a medium skillet, lightly sauté squash and onion in 1 tablespoon (15 milliliters) of the butter until onion is translucent. Add spaghetti sauce and season with salt and pepper; simmer 5 minutes and set aside. Beat together the eggs and water. In a large skillet, scramble eggs in remaining butter. Serve eggs topped with vegetable-sauce mixture.

> **Yield:** 4 servings
> **Exchange:** (1 serving) 1 bread, 1 vegetable, 1 medium-fat meat, 1 fat
> **Calories:** (1 serving) 213

SCRAMBLED EGGS PRIMAVERA

2 tablespoons	Mazola corn oil	30 milliliters
1 cup	zucchini (chopped)	250 milliliters
¹/₂ cup	mushrooms (sliced)	125 milliliters
¹/₄ cup	green onion (thinly sliced)	60 milliliters
4	eggs (lightly beaten with fork)	4
dash	dried basil	dash
4	English muffins (split & toasted)	4
1	tomato (chopped)	1
1 tablespoon	parsley	15 milliliters

In a skillet, heat oil over medium-high heat. Add next 3 ingredients. Cook and stir for 2 minutes or until zucchini is crisp-tender. Reduce heat to medium low. Add eggs and basil. Cook and stir for 3 to 4 minutes or until eggs are set. Spoon onto muffin halves. Garnish with tomato and parsley.

> **Yield:** 4 servings
> **Exchange:** (1 serving) 2 bread, 1 low-fat milk, 1 vegetable
> **Calories:** (1 serving) 290

"A Diet for the Young at Heart" by Mazola.

BAKED APPLES

4 medium	Rome apples	4 medium
¹/₄ cup	walnuts (chopped)	60 milliliters
¹/₄ cup	raisins	60 milliliters
¹/₄ cup	Health Valley Orangeola cereal with almonds & dates	60 milliliters
¹/₄ teaspoon	ground cinnamon	1 milliliter

Wash and core apples. Place in ovenproof dish. In small bowl, mix together the remaining ingredients. Divide into 4 portions and fill each apple hole with 1 portion. Cover and bake at 350°F (175°C) for 1 hour.

Yield: 4 servings
Exchange: (1 serving) ¹/₂ bread, 2 fruit, 1 fat
Calories: (1 serving) 165

From Health Valley Foods.

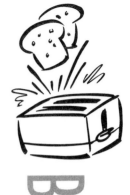

BREAKFAST

BAKED APPLE FRITTERS

1 cup	Health Valley honey graham crackers (crushed into crumbs)	250 milliliters
1 teaspoon	ground cinnamon	5 milliliters
2 large	pippin apples (cored & each sliced into 4 rings)	2 large
4 tablespoons	lemon juice	60 milliliters

Combine graham cracker crumbs with cinnamon. Dip apple slices in lemon juice and then graham cracker crumbs. Coat well on both sides. Place on greased cookie sheet. Bake at 400°F (200°C) for 15 to 20 minutes.

Yield: 4 servings
Exchange: (1 serving) 2 bread, 1 fruit
Calories: (1 serving) 170

From Health Valley Foods.

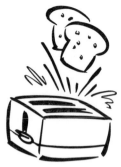

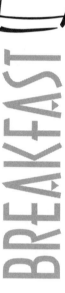

FRIED APPLE FRITTERS

2	large apples	2
1 cup	all-purpose flour	250 milliliters
1/2 cup	skim milk	125 milliliters
2 teaspoons	baking powder	10 milliliters
1/4 teaspoon	salt	1 milliliter
1	egg (beaten)	1
	vegetable oil for frying	

Core, peel, and slice the apples into 16 sections each. Combine remaining ingredients in a bowl and beat until smooth. Dip each apple slice into the batter. Heat the oil to 365°F (184°C). Fry apple sections until golden brown; drain on paper towels. You can fry 3 or 4 fritters at a time in a saucepan; do not overfill the saucepan with oil.) Serve hot.

Yield: 32 fritters
Exchange: (1 fritter) 1/4 bread
Calories: (1 fritter) 19
Carbohydrates: (1 fritter) 4 grams

WHEAT GERM WAFFLES

1 3/4 cups	sifted Stone-Buhr all-purpose flour	440 milliliters
3 tablespoons	granulated sugar replacement	45 milliliters
2 teaspoons	baking powder	10 milliliters
	salt	
2/3 cup	Stone-Buhr wheat-germ	160 milliliters
2 cups	skim milk	500 milliliters
1/3 cup	vegetable oil	90 milliliters
2	eggs (separated)	2

Sift together the flour, sugar replacement, baking powder and salt. Add wheat germ and stir to mix. Combine and beat milk, oil and egg yolks. Add to flour mixture; beat until smooth. In another bowl, beat egg whites until stiff but not dry. Fold into batter. Bake in preheated waffle iron.

Yield: 5 servings
Exchange: (1 serving) 2 bread, 1 low-fat milk
Calories: (1 serving) 261

Based on a recipe of Arnold Foods Company, Inc.

CRISPY WAFFLES

2	eggs (separated)	2
2 teaspoons	baking powder	10 milliliters
1/4 teaspoon	salt	1 milliliter
1 tablespoon	granulated sugar replacement	15 milliliters
1 cup	skim milk	250 milliliters
3 tablespoons	vegetable oil	45 milliliters
1 1/3 cups	all-purpose flour	340 milliliters

Beat egg whites in a bowl until stiff. Beat egg yolks, baking powder, salt, and sugar replacement in another bowl. Gradually add the milk and oil to the yolks alternately with the flour; beat until smooth. Fold in the beaten egg whites. Bake in a preheated waffle iron, according to the manufacturer's directions.

Yield: 4 large waffles or 8 servings
Exchange: (1 serving) 1 1/2 bread
Calories: (1 serving) 113
Carbohydrates: (1 serving) 17 grams

BUTTERMILK WAFFLES

1/2 cup	all-purpose flour	125 milliliters
1/2 cup	dry oatmeal	125 milliliters
1/4 cup	yellow cornmeal	60 milliliters
1 tablespoon	baking powder	15 milliliters
2 teaspoons	Butter Buds natural butter-flavored mix	10 milliliters
1/4 teaspoon	salt	1 milliliter
1	egg	1
1/4 cup	low-calorie margarine (melted & cooled)	60 milliliters
1 1/2 cups	buttermilk	375 milliliters

Combine the flour, oatmeal, cornmeal, baking powder, Butter Buds, and salt in a medium bowl. Add the egg and margarine; stir to mix. Stir in the buttermilk. Cover and allow the batter to rest 20 to 30 minutes or until doubled in size. Bake waffles in a preheated waffle iron, according to the manufacturer's directions.

Yield: 6 large waffles or 12 servings
Exchange: (1 serving) 1 bread
Calories: (1 serving) 79
Carbohydrates: (1 serving) 14 grams

BREAKFAST

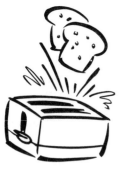

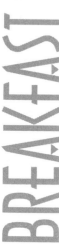

BREAKFAST

FRENCH TOAST

2	eggs (beaten)	2
2/3 cup	skim milk	180 milliliters
1/4 teaspoon	salt	1 milliliter
8 slices	bread	8 slices

Combine eggs, milk, and salt in flat dish; stir with a fork to blend. Lay each piece of bread into the egg mixture and turn over. Fry on a lightly greased griddle or skillet.

Yield: 8 servings
Exchange: (1 serving) 1 bread, 1/3 medium-fat meat
Calories: (1 serving) 102
Carbohydrates: (1 serving) 15 grams

CRISPY BAKED FRENCH TOAST

2	eggs (well-beaten)	2
1/2 cup	2% milk	125 milliliters
1/2 teaspoon	salt	2 milliliters
1/2 teaspoon	vanilla	2 milliliters
6 slices	Oroweat Northridge bread	6 slices
1 cup	Stone-Buhr bran flakes	250 milliliters
1/4 cup	margarine (melted)	60 milliliters

Combine eggs, milk, salt and vanilla in shallow dish or pan. Dip bread in egg mixture, turning once; allow time for both sides to absorb liquid. Coat evenly with bran flakes and place in a single layer on a well-greased baking sheet. Drizzle with the margarine. Bake at 450°F (230°C) for about 10 minutes or until crisp and browned. Serve warm.

Yield: 6 servings
Exchange: (1 serving) 1 1/2 bread, 2 fat
Calories: (1 serving) 192

With the compliments of Arnold Foods Company, Inc.

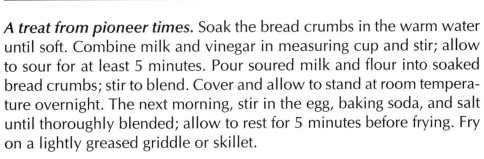

OLD-STYLE FLANNEL PANCAKES

2 cups	dry bread crumbs	500 milliliters
1 cup	warm water	250 milliliters
2 cups	skim milk	500 milliliters
1 tablespoon	cider vinegar	15 milliliters
1 cup	all-purpose flour	250 milliliters
1	egg (beaten)	1
1 teaspoon	baking soda	5 milliliters
1/2 teaspoon	salt	2 milliliters

A treat from pioneer times. Soak the bread crumbs in the warm water until soft. Combine milk and vinegar in measuring cup and stir; allow to sour for at least 5 minutes. Pour soured milk and flour into soaked bread crumbs; stir to blend. Cover and allow to stand at room temperature overnight. The next morning, stir in the egg, baking soda, and salt until thoroughly blended; allow to rest for 5 minutes before frying. Fry on a lightly greased griddle or skillet.

Yield: 20 servings
Exchange: (1 serving) 1 bread
Calories: (1 serving) 70
Carbohydrates: (1 serving) 13 grams

BRAN PANCAKES

1 cup	all-purpose flour	250 milliliters
2 teaspoons	baking powder	10 milliliters
1/2 teaspoon	salt	2 milliliters
2 teaspoons	granulated sugar replacement	10 milliliters
1/2 cup	bran cereal	125 milliliters
1 cup	skim milk (warmed)	250 milliliters
1	egg	1
2 tablespoons	vegetable oil	30 milliliters

In a medium bowl, mix and sift together the flour, baking powder, salt, and sugar replacement. Stir in the bran. Slowly add the skim milk and stir to blend. Beat in the egg. Add the oil and mix thoroughly. (Add a small amount of water, if batter is too thick.) Fry on a lightly greased hot griddle or skillet.

Yield: 10 servings
Exchange: (1 serving) 1 bread
Calories: (1 serving) 79
Carbohydrates: (1 serving) 13 grams

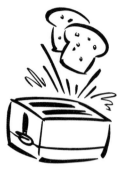

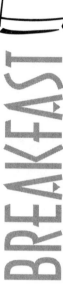

BREAKFAST

SESAME WHOLE WHEAT PANCAKES

1 cup	Stone-Buhr whole wheat pancake mix	250 milliliters
1¼ cups	skim milk	310 milliliters
1	egg	1
⅓ cup	Stone-Buhr sesame seeds (toasted)	90 milliliters

Combine the pancake mix, milk and egg. Pour a little less than ¼ cup (60 milliliters) batter for each pancake onto a lightly greased griddle. Immediately sprinkle each pancake with about 2 teaspoons (10 milliliters) toasted sesame seeds. Turn pancake when bubbles appear on the surface.

Yield: 6 servings
Exchange: (1 serving) 1 bread, 1 medium-fat meat
Calories: (1 serving) 150

With the compliments of Arnold Foods Company, Inc.

SWEET CORNMEAL PANCAKES

1	egg	1
1¼ cups	skim milk	310 milliliters
1 tablespoon	dietetic maple syrup	15 milliliters
¼ cup	solid vegetable shortening (melted)	60 milliliters
1 cup	all-purpose flour	250 milliliters
2 teaspoons	baking powder	10 milliliters
1 teaspoon	salt	5 milliliters
½ teaspoon	baking soda	2 milliliters
½ cup	yellow cornmeal	125 milliliters

In a medium bowl, beat together the egg, skim milk, syrup, and melted shortening. In another bowl, sift together the flour, baking powder, salt, and baking soda. Add to the egg mixture and beat until smooth. Stir in the cornmeal just until blended. Fry on a lightly greased nonstick griddle or skillet over medium heat.

Yield: 16 servings
Exchange: (1 serving) ¾ bread
Calories: (1 serving) 52
Carbohydrates: (1 serving) 12 grams

BUCKWHEAT PANCAKES

¹/₂ cup	dry bread crumbs	125 milliliters
2¹/₂ cups	skim milk (scalded)	625 milliliters
¹/₂ teaspoon	salt	2 milliliters
1¹/₂ teaspoons	dry yeast	7 milliliters
2 cups	buckwheat flour	500 milliliters
2 tablespoons	dietetic maple syrup	30 milliliters
¹/₄ teaspoon	baking soda	1 milliliter
2 tablespoons	warm water	30 milliliters

Place bread crumbs in a large bowl. Pour hot milk over the crumbs; stir in the salt and allow to cool to lukewarm. Then add the yeast and stir to dissolve. Add the buckwheat flour and stir until smooth. Cover and store in a warm place overnight. The next morning, add the dietetic syrup, baking soda, and warm water; beat until smooth. (Add a small amount of extra water, if batter is too thick.) Fry on a lightly greased hot griddle or skillet.

> **Yield:** 20 servings
> **Exchange:** (1 serving) ³/₄ bread
> **Calories:** (1 serving) 53
> **Carbohydrates:** (1 serving) 10 grams

KIDDY PANCAKES

1	egg	1
2 teaspoons	baking powder	10 milliliters
1 cup	all-purpose flour	250 milliliters
¹/₄ teaspoon	salt	1 milliliter
1 cup	skim milk	250 milliliters
2 tablespoons	vegetable oil	30 milliliters
	food coloring of your choice	

In a bowl, beat egg thoroughly. Add the remaining ingredients and beat until smooth. Color the batter as you wish. Fry on a lightly greased hot griddle or skillet. Optional: Pour batter into shapes for extra treats.

> **Yield:** 12 servings
> **Exchange:** (1 serving) ¹/₂ bread
> **Calories:** (1 serving) 35
> **Carbohydrates:** (1 serving) 7 grams

BREAKFAST

BAKED PANCAKES

3	eggs	3
1/2 cup	all-purpose flour (sifted)	125 milliliters
1/2 teaspoon	salt	2 milliliters
1/2 cup	skim milk	125 milliliters
2 tablespoons	low-calorie margarine (melted)	30 milliliters

Using a fork or wire beater, beat eggs in a bowl until well blended. In a small bowl, sift the flour and salt together. Gradually add flour mixture to eggs, beating after every addition. Add the milk and margarine, beating only slightly after each addition. Pour batter into a well-greased 10-inch (25-centimeter) skillet or baking dish. Bake at 450°F (230°C) for 20 minutes; reduce heat to 350°F (175°C) and continue for 10 more minutes. Slip out onto a heated serving platter. Serve immediately.

Yield: 8 servings
Exchange: (1 serving) 1/2 bread, 1/2 medium-fat meat
Calories: (1 serving) 73
Carbohydrates: (1 serving) 6 grams

FRENCH PANCAKES

3/4 cup	all-purpose flour	190 milliliters
1/8 teaspoon	salt	1/2 milliliter
1 teaspoon	baking powder	5 milliliters
1/2 cup	skim milk	125 milliliters

These pancakes are similar to crepes. Sift together the flour, salt, and baking powder. Slowly add the milk and beat until smooth. Fry on a lightly greased griddle or skillet.

Yield: 10 servings
Exchange: (1 serving) 1/2 bread
Calories: (1 serving) 35
Carbohydrates: (1 serving) 7 grams

FRESH BLUEBERRY PANCAKES

1	egg	1
1 cup	skim milk	250 milliliters
1 cup	all-purpose flour	250 milliliters
2 teaspoons	baking powder	10 milliliters
¼ teaspoon	salt	1 milliliter
½ cup	blueberries	125 milliliters

Beat the egg in a bowl until light. Add the skim milk. In a small bowl, mix together the flour, baking powder, and salt. Beat into the egg-milk mixture until smooth. Cover and allow to rest for 5 minutes. Fold in the blueberries. Fry on a slightly greased hot griddle or skillet.

Yield:	10 servings
Exchange:	(1 serving) 1 bread
Calories:	(1 serving) 67
Carbohydrates:	(1 serving) 12 grams

RASPBERRY PRESERVES

1 cup	fresh or frozen unsweetened raspberries	250 milliliters
1 teaspoon	low-cal pectin	5 milliliters
1 teaspoon	granulated sugar replacement	5 milliliters

Place raspberries in top of double boiler and cook over boiling water until soft and juicy. As they cook, crush berries against sides of double boiler. Add pectin and sugar replacement. Blend in thoroughly. Cook until medium thick.

Microwave: Place raspberries in glass bowl. Cook on HIGH for 4 minutes until soft and juicy. Add pectin and sugar replacement. Blend thoroughly. Cook on HIGH for 30 seconds.

Yield:	⅔ cup (180 milliliters)
Exchange:	(2 tablespoons/30 milliliters) ⅕ fruit
Calories:	(2 tablespoons/30 milliliters) 7

BREAKFAST

BREAKFAST

RAISIN-APPLE SPIRAL

1 package	active dry yeast	1 package
³/₄ cup	milk (warmed)	190 milliliters
¹/₄ cup	margarine (softened)	60 milliliters
¹/₂ teaspoon	salt	2 milliliters
2¹/₄ cups	all-purpose flour	560 milliliters
1 cup	wheat germ	250 milliliters
1	egg	1
1 recipe	Raisin Apple Filling (recipe follows)	1 recipe
	vegetable oil for brushing dough	
1	egg	1
1 tablespoon	water	15 milliliters
¹/₃ cup	Powdered Sugar Replacement	90 milliliters
	(recipe follows)	
¹/₄ teaspoon	orange rind (grated)	1 milliliter
3 teaspoons	orange juice	15 milliliters

In a large bowl, dissolve the yeast in warm milk. Add margarine and salt, stirring until margarine almost melts. Stir in 1 cup (250 milliliters) of the flour, wheat germ and egg. With an electric mixer, beat at medium speed for 2 minutes. Scrape bowl occasionally. With wooden spoon, gradually stir in just enough remaining flour to make a soft dough which leaves sides of bowl. Cover and allow to rise in warm, draft-free place about 1 hour or until doubled. Roll on floured board into a 24 x 4-inch (60 x 10-centimeter) strip. Spread the Raisin Apple Filling across middle of strip. To seal, lift dough and pinch lengthwise edges together with seam-side down, coil loosely, snail fashion. Place on greased baking sheet with space between to allow for rising. Brush dough lightly with oil. Cover and allow to rise about 1 hour or until doubled. Brush with 1 egg mixed with the water just before baking. Bake at 350°F (175°C) for 20 to 25 minutes until golden. Immediately remove from baking sheet. Cool slightly on rack. Combine powdered sugar replacement and orange rind and gradually add orange juice, beating until smooth. Drizzle on bread. Serve warm.

RAISIN-APPLE FILLING

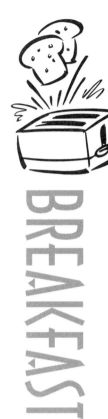

1 cup	apple (chopped)	250 milliliters
¹/₂ cup	raisins	125 milliliters
2 tablespoons	butter	30 milliliters
¹/₂ cup	walnuts (chopped)	125 milliliters
2 tablespoons	orange rind (grated)	30 milliliters
¹/₄ teaspoon	ground cinnamon	1 milliliter
¹/₄ teaspoon	ground or grated nutmeg	1 milliliter
dash	ground cloves	dash
dash	salt	dash

Combine apple, raisins and butter in a small saucepan. Cover and simmer over low heat for 10 minutes. Remove from heat and stir in the remaining ingredients. Cool.

Yield: 1 coffee cake or 24 servings
Exchange: (1 serving) 1 bread, 1 fat
Calories: (1 serving) 112

POWDERED SUGAR REPLACEMENT

2 cups	nonfat dry milk powder	500 milliliters
2 cups	cornstarch	500 milliliters
1 cup	granulated sugar replacement	250 milliliters

Combine all ingredients in food processor or blender. Whip until well blended into a powder.

Yield: 4 cups (1 kilogram)
Exchange: (1 serving–¹/₄ cup/60 milliliters) 1 bread or ¹/₂ nonfat milk, ¹/₂ bread
Calories: (1 serving–¹/₄ cup/60 milliliters) 81

SUNSHINE STOLLEN

2 inch	vanilla bean (split)	5 centimeters
1 cup	granulated sugar replacement	250 milliliters
2¹/₃ cups	all-purpose flour	585 milliliters
2 teaspoons	baking powder	10 milliliters
¹/₂ teaspoon	salt	2 milliliters
¹/₄ teaspoon	ground mace	1 milliliter
¹/₄ teaspoon	ground cardamom	1 milliliter
¹/₃ cup	almonds (ground)	90 milliliters
¹/₂ cup	low-calorie margarine	125 milliliters
1 cup	low-fat cottage cheese	250 milliliters
1	egg	1
2 tablespoons	water	30 milliliters
¹/₂ teaspoon	vanilla extract	2 milliliters
¹/₂ teaspoon	rum flavoring	2 milliliters
¹/₃ cup	currants	90 milliliters
¹/₃ cup	raisins	90 milliliters
¹/₄ cup	lemon peel	60 milliliters
2 tablespoons	low-calorie margarine (melted)	30 milliliters

Note: Make the vanilla sugar replacement at least 3 days before you plan to make the stollen.

Vanilla sugar replacement: Bury the split vanilla bean in 1 cup (250 milliliters) of granulated sugar replacement in a container. Cover the container tightly. Allow vanilla bean to flavor sugar replacement for at least 3 days at room temperature.

Sunshine stollen: Combine ¹/₂ cup (125 milliliters) of the vanilla sugar replacement, flour, baking powder, salt, mace, cardamom, and almonds. Cut margarine into the mixture until it resembles coarse crumbs. Blend cottage cheese in a blender until smooth; pour into the flour mixture. Add the egg, water, vanilla, rum flavoring, currants, raisins, and lemon peel; stir to thoroughly mix. Form the dough into a ball. Knead on a lightly floured surface 10 to 12 times or until dough is smooth. Roll dough into an 8 x 10-inch (20 x 25-centimeter) oval. With the back of your hand, crease the dough just off the middle, parallel to the 10-inch (25-centimeter) side; fold the smaller section over the larger. Brush with half of the melted margarine. Bake on an ungreased baking sheet at 350°F (175°C) for 45 minutes or until done. Remove stollen from oven and allow to cool. Brush with the remaining melted margarine and sprinkle with 2 tablespoons (30 milliliters) of the granulated vanilla sugar replacement.

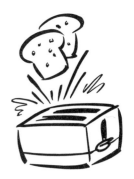

Yield: 20 servings
Exchange: (1 serving) 1 bread, ³/₄ fat
Calories: (1 serving) 106
Carbohydrates: (1 serving) 15 grams

PLAIN YEAST KUCHEN DOUGH

1 package	dry yeast	1 package
¹/₄ cup	lukewarm water	60 milliliters
1³/₄ cups	skim milk (scalded)	440 milliliters
¹/₂ cup	granulated sugar replacement	125 milliliters
¹/₄ cup	low-calorie margarine	60 milliliters
¹/₄ cup	butter	60 milliliters
1 tablespoon	lemon peel (freshly grated)	15 milliliters
1 teaspoon	salt	5 milliliters
1	egg (beaten)	1
6 cups	all-purpose flour	1¹/₂ liters

To make the dough, dissolve the yeast in lukewarm water. In a bowl, combine the scalded milk, sugar replacement, margarine, butter, lemon peel, and salt; stir and cool to lukewarm. When cooled, beat in the egg. Stir in the yeast mixture. Add enough flour to make a soft dough (about 3 cups or 750 milliliters). Turn out on floured surface and knead in remaining flour until smooth and elastic. Cover tightly and allow to rise until double in size. Punch down and use as directed in recipe or form into desired shapes.

This dough can also be made into doughnuts and fried. To bake the kuchen, place on a well-greased baking sheet or 2 large pans. Bake at 375°F (190°C) until browned; baking time will vary, depending on size of loaves.

Yield: 32 servings
Exchange: (1 serving) 1 bread, ³/₄ fat
Calories: (1 serving) 107
Carbohydrates: (1 serving) 17 grams

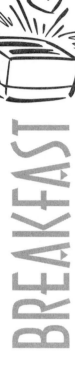

STRAWBERRY KUCHEN

Crust:	**1 cup**	all-purpose flour	250 milliliters
	1/2 cup	low-calorie margarine	125 milliliters
	1	egg yolk	1
	1 tablespoon	liquid sweetener	15 milliliters
Filling:	**2 cups**	strawberries (sliced)	500 milliliters
	2	eggs (beaten)	2
	1/4 cup	granulated sugar relacement	60 milliliters
	2 teaspoons	all-purpose flour	10 milliliters

Crust: Combine ingredients in a food processor or bowl. Cut into small pea-sized crumbs. Pat tightly into the bottom of a 13 x 9-inch (33 x 23-centimeter) pan.

Filling: Combine all filling ingredients in a bowl; stir to blend. Allow to rest for 10 minutes; then stir again. Pour into the crust and spread evenly. Bake at 350°F (175°C) for 35 to 40 minutes or until filling is set.

Yield:	12 servings
Exchange:	(1 serving) 2/3 bread, 1 fat
Calories:	(1 serving) 100
Carbohydrates:	(1 serving) 10 grams

SUPERB APPLE COFFEECAKE

1/2 recipe	Plain Yeast Kuchen Dough (page 27)	1/2 recipe
1/3 cup	dietetic maple syrup	90 milliliters
2	apples	2

Pour dietetic maple syrup into bottom of a well-oiled 8-inch (20-centimeter) baking pan. Peel and slice apples over the syrup. Punch down and roll the dough into an 8-inch (20-centimeter) square. Cover apples in the pan with the dough. Using your fingers, push dough to the sides and corners of the pan. Cover and allow to rise until double in size. Bake at 350°F (175°C) for 30 to 35 minutes or until done and brown. Immediately turn upside down onto a serving dish. Cut into 2-inch (5-centimeter) squares.

Yield:	16 servings
Exchange:	(1 serving) 1 bread, 3/4 fat, 1/4 fruit
Calories:	(1 serving) 111
Carbohydrates:	(1 serving) 19 grams

TOASTED COCONUT COFFEECAKE

1/2 **recipe**	Plain Yeast Kuchen Dough (page 27)	1/2 recipe
1/3 **cup**	unsweetened coconut flakes	90 milliliters
1 **tablespoon**	granulated brown sugar replacement	15 milliliters
1 **tablespoon**	granulated sugar replacement	15 milliliters
1 **teaspoon**	lemon peel	5 milliliters
1/4 **teaspoon**	ground cinnamon	1 milliliter
1/8 **teaspoon**	ground nutmeg	1/2 milliliter

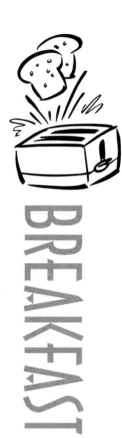

Pull dough into an 18-inch (45-centimeter)-long strip; set aside. Place coconut in a small skillet. Over low heat, flip and fry coconut until it is browned and toasted. Sprinkle coconut over bottom of a well-greased tube pan. In a bowl, combine the brown and granulated sugar replacements, lemon peel, cinnamon, and nutmeg. Sprinkle over coconut in skillet. Place dough strip over entire mixture. With your fingers, work dough to sides of the pan. Cover and allow to rise until double in size. Bake at 350°F (175°C) for 30 to 40 minutes or until done. Turn upside down onto a serving dish.

Yield:	16 servings
Exchange:	(1 serving) 1 bread, 1 fat
Calories:	(1 serving) 113
Carbohydrates:	(1 serving) 17 grams

PRUNE STREUSEL COFFEECAKE

3 tablespoons	all-purpose flour	45 milliliters
2 tablespoons	granulated brown sugar replacement	30 milliliters
2 teaspoons	ground cinnamon	10 milliliters
1/2 **cup**	Bran Buds cereal	125 milliliters
3 tablespoons	margarine (softened)	45 milliliters
1 cup	all-purpose flour	250 milliliters
3/4 **teaspoon**	baking powder	4 milliliters
3/4 **teaspoon**	baking soda	4 milliliters
1/2 **teaspoon**	salt	2 milliliters
1/2 **teaspoon**	ground cinnamon	2 milliliters
3/4 **cup**	Bran Buds cereal	190 milliliters
1/2 **cup**	margarine (softened)	125 milliliters
2 tablespoons	granulated sugar replacement	30 milliliters
2	eggs	2
1 cup	plain low-fat yogurt	250 milliliters
1/2 **cup**	pitted prunes (finely cut)	125 milliliters

Topping: Measure the first 5 ingedients into a small mixing bowl. Mix with fork or fingers until crumbly. Set aside.

Cake: Stir together 1 cup (250 milliliters) flour, baking powder, baking soda, salt, cinnamon and 3/4 cup (190 milliliters) cereal. Set aside. In a large bowl, beat 1/2 cup (125 milliliters) margarine and sugar replacement until well blended. Add eggs. Beat well. Stir in yogurt. Add flour mixture, mixing thoroughly. Spread half the batter evenly in greased 9-inch (23-centimeter) square baking pan. Sprinkle evenly over the batter, half the prunes and then, half the topping. Spread remaining batter over the top and sprinkle batter with the remaining prunes and topping mixture. Bake at 350°F (175°C) about 40 minutes or until done. Serve warm.

Yield:	16 servings
Exchange:	(1 serving) 1 bread, 2/3 low-fat milk, 1/2 fat
Calories:	(1 serving) 180

Adapted from a recipe from Kellogg's Test Kitchens.

CRUMB COFFEECAKE

2 cups	all-purpose flour	500 milliliters
3/4 **cup**	granulated sugar relacement	190 milliliters
1/2 **teaspoon**	ground cinnamon	2 milliliters
1/2 **teaspoon**	ground ginger	2 milliliters
1/4 **teaspoon**	ground nutmeg	1 milliliter
1/2 **cup**	low-calorie margarine	125 milliliters
1/3 **cup**	raisins	90 milliliters
1/3 **cup**	walnuts (chopped)	90 milliliters
1	egg (beaten)	1
3/4 **cup**	buttermilk	190 milliliters
1 teaspoon	baking powder	5 milliliters
1/2 **teaspoon**	baking soda	2 milliliters

Sift the flour twice. In a bowl, combine the sifted flour, sugar replacement, cinnamon, ginger, and nutmeg. Cut in the margarine until the mixture forms crumbs. Remove 1 cup (250 milliliters) of the mixture and reserve. Stir the raisins and walnuts into the remaining crumb mixture. In another bowl, mix together the egg, buttermilk, baking powder, and baking soda. Stir into the flour mixture just until mixed. Spread half of the reserved crumbs on the bottom of a well-greased 8-inch (20 centimeter) square baking pan. Pour the batter over the crumbs and spread evenly. Sprinkle with the remaining crumbs. Bake at 375°F (190°C) for 40 minutes or until done. Cool in the pan.

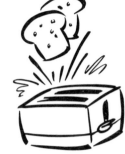

Yield:	16 servings
Exchange:	(1 serving) 1 bread, ³/₄ fat
Calories:	(1 serving) 107
Carbohydrates:	(1 serving) 13 grams

BLUEBERRY YOGURT COFFEECAKE

1 package	dry yeast	1 package
¹/₄ cup	lukewarm water	60 milliliters
¹/₃ cup	skim milk	90 milliliters
8 ounces	blueberry low-calorie yogurt	240 grams
1¹/₄ teaspoons	granulated fructose	6 milliliters
2³/₄ cups	all-purpose flour	690 milliliters

Dissolve the yeast in warm water; set aside. Scald the skim milk in a medium saucepan. Add the yogurt and stir to dissolve. Stir in the fructose. Allow to cool to lukewarm. When lukewarm, stir in yeast mixture. In the same saucepan, stir in 1 cup (250 milliliters) of the flour. Beat until smooth. Gradually add remaining flour. Cover and allow to rise for 1¹/₂ hours. Turn out onto board and knead until smooth and elastic. (Dough will be soft.) Form into a ball and wrap tightly in plastic. Place in refrigerator overnight. (You might have to punch dough down a second time and rewrap in plastic.) When ready to bake, place dough on a lightly floured surface; cut in half. Roll each half into a small square to fit an 8-inch (20-centimeter) pan. Place dough in two lightly greased 8-inch (20-centimeter) square pans. Push dough to edges; using your finger, push a small ridge up the sides. Cover and allow to rise until over double in size. Bake at 350°F (175°C) for 25 to 30 minutes or until done.

Yield:	2 coffeecakes or 32 servings
Exchange:	(1 serving) ¹/₂ bread
Calories:	(1 serving) 29
Carbohydrates:	(1 serving) 9 grams

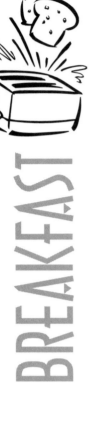

GOLDEN CORN COINS

1 cup	yellow cornmeal	250 milliliters
1 teaspoon	salt	5 milliliters
	boiling water	

This is strictly for the family when speed is needed. Heat the oven to 450°F (230°C). Place a well-greased, rimmed cookie sheet in the oven. Combine the cornmeal, salt, and just enough boiling water to make a thick pancake-like batter. Carefully remove greased sheet from oven. Using a large serving spoon, quickly spoon batter onto the hot grease in 36 large fifty-cent-size rounds. Place in oven and bake for 10 to 15 minutes or until lightly browned. Serve hot.

Yield: 36 coins
Exchange: (1 coin) ⅕ bread
Calories: (1 coin) 13
Carbohydrates: (1 coin) 3 grams

IRISH SCONES

2 cups	all-purpose flour	500 milliliters
½ cup	solid vegetable shortening	125 milliliters
1 teaspoon	baking soda	5 milliliters
1 teaspoon	cream of tartar	5 milliliters
¼ teaspoon	salt	1 milliliter
⅓ cup	currants	90 milliliters
¾ cup	skim milk	190 milliliters

In a food processor or bowl, combine the flour, shortening, baking soda, cream of tartar, and salt; cut into coarse crumbs. Mix in the currants. (If using a food processor, transfer mixture to a bowl.) Pour all of the milk into the mixture. Using a fork, gently stir until the dough holds together. Form into a ball and knead 10 to 12 times. Roll on a lightly floured surface to make a ½-inch (1.3-centimetre)-thick circle. Cut into 10 wedges. Place wedges about 1 inch (2.5 centimeters) apart on an ungreased baking sheet. Bake at 400°F (200°C) for 12 to 15 minutes or until done.

Yield: 10 servings
Exchange: (1 serving) 1 bread, 2 fat, ½ fruit
Calories: (1 serving) 192
Carbohydrates: (1 serving) 22 grams

SPICY PRUNE BREAD

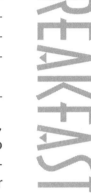

2 cups	all purpose flour (sifted)	500 milliliters
2¹/₂ teaspoons	baking powder	12 milliliters
¹/₂ teaspoon	baking soda	2 milliliters
1 teaspoon	salt	5 milliliters
1 teaspoon	ground cinnamon	5 milliliters
¹/₂ teaspoon	ground or grated nutmeg	2 milliliters
¹/₄ teaspoon	ground cloves	1 milliliter
1 cup	oatmeal	250 milliliters
1¹/₄ cups	buttermilk	310 milliliters
2 tablespoons	vegetable oil	30 milliliters
1 cup	prunes (cooked, drained, pitted & diced)	250 milliliters

Sift together the flour, baking powder, baking soda, salt, cinnamon, nutmeg and cloves. Stir in the oatmeal. Add buttermilk and oil; stir to completely blend. Fold in prunes. Spread into a well-greased 9 x 5-inch (23 x 13-centimeter) loaf pan. Bake at 350°F (175°C) for 1 hour or until done. Turn out on rack to cool.

> **Yield:** 1 loaf or 16 servings
> **Exchange:** (1 serving) 1 bread, ¹/₄ fruit
> **Calories:** (1 serving) 85

SWEET AND LOVELY DOUGHNUTS

1	frozen white bread dough (thawed)	1
3 tablespoons	granulated fructose	45 milliliters
	vegetable oil for frying	

These doughnuts are so easy to make. Roll the dough on an unfloured surface. Sprinkle dough with the fructose. Roll up as a jelly roll. Reroll dough on an unfloured surface into an 8-inch (20-centimeter) square. With a sharp knife, cut the dough into 12 equal pieces. Push your thumb into the middle of each piece. Form doughnut by turning each piece around with your fingers. Place on a lightly floured surface. Cover and allow to double in size. Heat the oil to 375°F (190°C). Drop in a few doughnuts at a time; turn frequently until puffed and golden. Remove with a slotted spoon and drain on paper towels.

> **Yield:** 12 doughnuts
> **Exchange:** (1 doughnut) 1¹/₂ bread
> **Calories:** (1 doughnut) 96
> **Carbohydrates:** (1 doughnut) 18 grams

BAKED ORANGE DOUGHNUTS

2 packages	yeast	2 packages
¹/₂ cup	warm water	125 milliliters
1 cup	orange juice	250 milliliters
¹/₃ cup	low-calorie margarine (melted & cooled)	90 milliliters
³/₄ cup	granulated sugar replacement	190 milliliters
2 teaspoons	salt	10 milliliters
1¹/₂ tablespoons	orange peel	22 milliliters
2	eggs	2
3 cups	all-purpose flour	750 milliliters
	vegetable cooking spray	

Dissolve the yeast in warm water; set aside until it starts to bubble. In a large bowl, combine the yeast mixture, orange juice, margarine, sugar replacement, salt, orange peel, eggs, and 2 cups (500 milliliters) of the flour; beat on high speed for about 4 minutes. Gradually beat in the remaining flour. Transfer dough to a lightly floured surface and knead until smooth and elastic. Place dough in an oiled bowl; cover and allow to rise until doubled in size. Punch dough down. Roll out on a lightly floured surface until ¹/₄ inch (6 millimeters) thick. Lift dough from surface and turn over; cover with a towel and allow to rest for 2 minutes. Cut dough with a doughnut cutter; place doughnuts on a greased baking sheet. Allow to rise until almost double in size. Bake at 350°F (175°C) for 10 minutes or until lightly browned. Coat immediately with the cooking spray.

Yield: 30 doughnuts
Exchange: (1 doughnut) 1 bread
Calories: (1 doughnut) 60
Carbohydrates: (1 doughnut) 11 grams

PARK DOUGHNUTS

3	eggs (separated)	3
³/₄ cup	granulated sugar replacement	190 milliliters
4¹/₂ cups	all-purpose flour	1¹/₈ liters
5 teaspoons	baking powder	25 milliliters
1¹/₂ teaspoons	salt	7 milliliters
1 cup	skim milk	250 milliliters
1 teaspoon	nutmeg	5 milliliters
3 tablespoons	vegetable oil	45 milliliters
	vegetable oil for frying	

In a bowl, beat the egg whites until stiff and dry. Beat the yolks into the egg whites, one at a time, until lemon colored. Gradually beat in the sugar replacement. In another bowl, sift flour, baking powder, and salt together twice. Add flour mixture alternately with the skim milk to the egg mixture, beating well after each addition. Add the nutmeg and the 3 tablespoons (45 milliliters) oil. Turn out onto a lightly floured surface. Roll until 1/2 inch (1.3 centimeter) thick and cut with doughnut cutter. Heat frying oil to 375°F (190°C). Drop in a few doughnuts at a time. Fry until puffed and golden brown. Remove with a slotted spoon and drain on paper towels.

Yield:	36 doughnuts
Exchange:	(1 doughnut) 1 bread
Calories:	(1 doughnut) 74
Carbohydrates:	(1 doughnut) 11 grams

RAISED CHERRY-YOGURT DOUGHNUTS

1 package	dry yeast	1 package
1/4 cup	lukewarm water	60 milliliters
1/3 cup	skim milk (scalded)	90 milliliters
8 ounces	cherry low-calorie yogurt	240 grams
1/4 teaspoon	cherry flavoring	1 milliliter
3 cups	all-purpose flour	750 milliliters
	vegetable oil for frying	

Dissolve the yeast in lukewarm water; set aside. Combine the scalded milk, yogurt, and cherry flavoring in a large bowl; beat to blend. Add yeast mixture and half of the flour and beat until soft. Add 3/4 cup (190 milliliters) more flour; mix until blended. Sprinkle remaining flour on a work surface. Knead dough on the floured surface until flour is incorporated and dough is smooth and elastic. Place in a greased bowl; turn once to coat both sides. Cover tightly with plastic. Refrigerate for 6 hours or overnight. Place dough on a very lightly floured surface. Roll until 1/2 inch (1.3 centimeter) thick. Cut with a doughnut cutter. Allow to rise for 30 to 45 minutes. Fry in vegetable oil that has been heated to 365°F (184°C). Turn and fry until lightly browned and done.

Yield:	18 doughnuts
Exchange:	(1 doughnut) 1 bread
Calories:	(1 doughnut) 82
Carbohydrates:	(1 doughnut) 19 grams

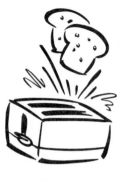

TOAST STICKS

6	white bread slices	6
2 tablespoons	low-calorie margarine (melted)	30 milliliters

Remove crusts from bread. Brush each piece with the melted margarine. Cut each piece into 3 equal pieces. Toast in hot oven at 400°F (200°C) for 8 minutes or until golden brown.

Yield: 18 servings
Exchange: (1 serving) ¹/₃ bread
Calories: (1 serving) 22
Carbohydrates: (1 serving) 4 grams

ORANGEOLA BARS

1¹/₄ cups	Health Valley Orangeola cereal	310 milliliters
¹/₄ cup	Health Valley Sprouts 7 cereal	60 milliliters
¹/₃ cup	walnuts (finely ground)	90 milliliters
2 tablespoons	fresh or dried coconut (grated)	30 milliliters
dash	ground or grated nutmeg	dash
2 tablespoons	clover honey	30 milliliters
¹/₂ teaspoon	vanilla	2 milliliters
2	egg whites (beaten until stiff)	2

In a mixing bowl, combine cereals, nuts, coconut and nutmeg. Add honey and vanilla and mix thoroughly (it might be necessary to use your hands to do this). Then fold in egg whites and allow mixture to stand 2 to 3 minutes. Spread or press into greased 11 x 6¹/₂ x 2-inch (28 x 16.5 x 5-centimeter) baking pan. Bake in preheated 275°F (135°C) oven for 20 minutes. Remove from oven. Cut into 20 to 24 bars and transfer immediately to glass or china plate to cool.

Yield: 20 bars
Exchange: (1 bar) ²/₃ bread
Calories: (1 bar) 50

From Health Valley Foods.

ORANGEY PINEAPPLE-NUT SQUARES

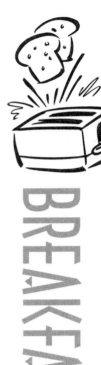

2 cups	Health Valley Orangeola cereal (finely crushed)	500 milliliters
1/2 teaspoon	ground ginger	2 milliliters
4	egg yolks	4
2 tablespoons	safflower oil	30 milliliters
3/4 cup	milk	190 milliliters
1/2 cup	pecans (chopped)	125 milliliters
1 cup	unsweetened crushed pineapple (drained)	250 milliliters
4	egg whites	4

In a medium bowl, combine cereal and ginger. In a small bowl, beat egg yolks, then add oil and milk. Add to dry ingredients, then stir in nuts and pineapple. Beat egg whites until stiff and fold them into batter. Spoon batter into greased 8-inch (20-centimeter)-square baking pan. Bake in preheated 350°F (175°C) oven for 30 to 35 minutes, until toothpick inserted in middle comes out dry.

Yield: 9 servings
Exchange: (1 serving) 2 bread, 1 fruit, 3 fat
Calories: (1 serving) 315

From Health Valley Foods.

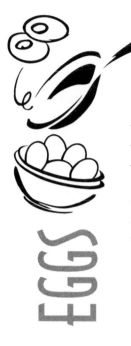

EGGS

SIMPLE BAKED EGG

1	egg	1
¹/₂ teaspoon	low-calorie margarine	2 milliliters
	salt & pepper to taste	

Melt margarine in a custard cup. Break egg into the cup. Sprinkle with salt and pepper. Bake at 350°F (175°C) for about 15 minutes or until the egg is firm but not hard. Serve hot.

Yield:	1 serving
Exchange:	1 medium-fat meat, ¹/₂ fat
Calories:	100
Carbohydrates:	negligible

EGGS À LA KING

2 tablespoons	butter	30 milliliters
3 tablespoons	all-purpose flour	45 milliliters
2 cups	skim milk	500 milliliters
	salt & pepper to taste	
6	eggs (hard-cooked)	6
3	small carrots (sliced & cooked)	3
¹/₃ cup	peas (cooked)	90 milliliters
¹/₃ cup	snow-capped mushrooms (sliced & cooked)	90 milliliters
1	medium pimiento (sliced & cooked)	1
	fresh parsley for garnish (optional)	
6	bread slices (toasted)	6

Melt butter in top of a double boiler. Blend in the flour; add the milk and stir until sauce thickens. Season with salt and pepper and cook 3 minutes longer. Slice or chop the eggs. Gently fold eggs, carrots, peas, and mushrooms into the sauce. Place toast on heated serving plates. Evenly divide egg mixture among the 6 pieces of toast. Arrange pimiento slices in crisscross fashion over the top of egg mixture. If desired, garnish plate with fresh parsley.

Yield:	6 servings
Exchange:	(1 serving) 1 medium-fat meat, 1¹/₂ bread
Calories:	(1 serving) 186
Carbohydrates:	(1 serving) 22 grams

BAKED EGG & CHEESE

1	egg	1
¹/₂ teaspoon	low-calorie margarine	2 milliliters
1 teaspoon	sharp Cheddar cheese (shredded)	5 milliliters

An easy alternative to an omelette. Melt margarine in a custard cup. Break egg into the cup and top with Cheddar cheese. Sprinkle with salt and pepper. Bake at 350°F (175°C) for 15 minutes or until the egg is firm and cheese is melted. Serve hot.

Yield: 1 serving
Exchange: 1 medium-fat meat, 1 fat
Calories: 122
Carbohydrates: negligible

EGGS WITH VEGETABLES

1	eggplant slice	1
2	tomato slices	2
1	egg	1
	salt & pepper to taste	
	fresh parsley for garnish	

An easy dish for a luncheon. Prepare this recipe for each serving. Sauté eggplant in a nonstick skillet; place eggplant on a heated serving dish in a warm oven. Sauté tomato slices in the skillet; arrange on the eggplant. Fry the egg to desired doneness; set over the tomato slices. Season with salt and pepper. Garnish with fresh parsley.

Yield: 1 serving
Exchange: (1 serving) 1 medium-fat meat, ¹/₂ vegetable
Calories: (1 serving) 92
Carbohydrates: (1 serving) 3 grams

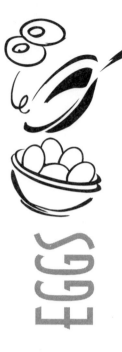

EGGS IN FLUFFY NESTS

4	eggs	4
	salt & pepper to taste	
4	hot toast slices	4
	paprika to taste	

This is really fun to make and fun to serve. Separate the eggs, leaving the yolk of each egg in its shell. Place whites in a bowl and season with salt and pepper. Beat until whites are stiff and form peaks. Heap onto toast slices. Make a hollow in the middle of each mound and gently slip egg yolk into the hollow. Sprinkle lightly with paprika. Bake at 350°F (175°C) for 10 to 12 minutes or until the yolks are slightly firm and whites are lightly browned.

Yield: 4 servings
Exchange: (1 serving) 1 bread, 1 medium-fat meat
Calories: (1 serving) 149
Carbohydrates: (1 serving) 15 grams

FRENCH-STYLE EGGS

1 tablespoon	butter	15 milliliters
3 tablespoons	all-purpose flour	45 milliliters
³/₄ cup	2 percent milk	190 milliliters
¹/₂ teaspoon	paprika	2 milliliters
¹/₄ teaspoon	salt	1 milliliter
dash	black pepper (freshly ground)	dash
6	eggs (hard-cooked)	6
¹/₄ cup	dry bread crumbs (finely ground)	60 milliliters
	vegetable oil for deep-fat frying	
¹/₂ cup	Quick Tomato Sauce (page 167)	125 milliliters

Melt butter in a saucepan; blend in the flour. Add milk and seasonings. Cook over low heat until sauce thickens, stirring constantly. Dip eggs in the sauce; cool eggs and roll in bread crumbs. Heat oil to 375°F (190°C). Fry eggs until brown. Serve hot with the tomato sauce.

Yield: 6 servings
Exchange: (1 serving) 1 bread, 1 medium-fat meat, 1 vegetable
Calories: (1 serving) 172
Carbohydrates: (1 serving) 19 grams

BACON & EGG CUP

1	bacon slice	1
1	egg	1
	black pepper to taste (freshly ground)	

Fry bacon in a skillet until almost crispy; cut into small pieces. Place in bottom and sides of a custard cup; break the egg into bacon-lined cup. Sprinkle with desired amount of pepper. Bake at 350°F (175°C) for 15 minutes or until egg is firm.

Yield:	1 serving
Exchange:	1$\frac{1}{2}$ medium-fat meat
Calories:	121
Carbohydrates:	negligible

EGG CROQUETTES

2 tablespoons	low-calorie margarine	30 milliliters
3 tablespoons	all-purpose flour	45 milliliters
$\frac{3}{4}$ cup	2 percent milk	190 milliliters
$\frac{1}{2}$ teaspoon	salt	2 milliliters
$\frac{1}{8}$ teaspoon	paprika	$\frac{1}{2}$ milliliter
4	eggs (hard-cooked)	4
1	raw egg	1
2 tablespoons	water	30 milliliters
$\frac{1}{3}$ cup	salted cracker crumbs	90 milliliters

Melt margarine in top of a double boiler; add the flour and stir constantly until blended. Add the milk, salt, and paprika. Cook and stir until mixture thickens. Chop the hard-cooked eggs; add to creamed mixture. Remove from heat and allow to cool. Combine the raw egg and water in small narrow bowl; beat until well blended. When egg/cream mixture is cold, shape into 6 large or 12 small croquettes. Roll in the cracker crumbs; then dip in egg-water and again in the crumbs. Refrigerate until completely chilled. Fry in deep fat, heated to 375°F (190°C), for about 3 to 5 minutes until golden brown. Serve hot.

Yield:	6 servings
Exchange:	(1 serving) 1 bread, 1 medium-fat meat
Calories:	(1 serving) 98
Carbohydrates:	(1 serving) 16 grams

EGGS IN TOMATO NESTS

4	tomatoes	4
4	eggs	4
4 teaspoons	butter	20 milliliters
	salt & pepper to taste	

Cut tops from tomatoes. Scoop out a hollow in the middle of each tomato large enough to hold the egg. Place 1 teaspoon (5 milliliters) of butter in each tomato hollow. Break an egg into each hollow. Place tomatoes on a baking sheet or 8 or 9-inch (20-or 23-centimetre) pie pan. Bake at 350°F (175°C) for 15 to 18 minutes or until eggs are firm and tomato is cooked.

Yield:	4 servings
Exchange:	(1 serving) 1 medium-fat meat, 1 vegetable, 1 fat
Calories:	(1 serving) 150
Carbohydrates:	(1 serving) 6 grams

EGGS, NEW ORLEANS STYLE

5	tomatoes (peeled & chopped)	5
$^1/_2$	green pepper (chopped)	$^1/_2$
$^1/_2$ cup	celery (chopped)	125 milliliters
$^1/_4$ cup	white onion (chopped)	60 milliliters
1	bay leaf	1
$^1/_2$ teaspoon	salt	2 milliliters
$^1/_4$ teaspoon	black pepper (freshly ground)	1 milliliter
$^3/_4$ cup	fine bread crumbs	190 milliliters
6	eggs	6
$^1/_2$ cup	American cheese (grated)	125 milliliters

In a saucepan, combine the tomatoes, green pepper, celery, onion, bay leaf, salt, and pepper. Cook and stir over medium heat for 10 minutes. Remove bay leaf. Stir in the bread crumbs. Spread the mixture into a lightly oiled casserole. With the back of a spoon, make 6 small hollows in the mixture and break the eggs into the hollows. Sprinkle with cheese. Bake at 350°F (175°C) for 15 to 20 minutes until eggs are firm and cheese has melted. Serve hot.

Yield:	6 servings
Exchange:	(1 serving) 1$^1/_2$ medium-fat meat, $^3/_4$ bread, 1 vegetable
Calories:	(1 serving) 190
Carbohydrates:	(1 serving) 16 grams

MUSHROOM-CAPPED EGGS

6	eggs (hard-cooked)	6
12	mushroom caps	12
1 cup	mushroom soup	250 milliliters
1 teaspoon	paprika	5 milliliters
1/2 teaspoon	salt	2 milliliters
	black pepper (freshly ground)	

These eggs have a pixie look that children love. Cut eggs in half. Place a mushroom cap on top of the yolk. Arrange mushroom-capped eggs in a single layer in a baking pan. Top with the soup. Sprinkle with paprika, salt and pepper. Bake at 350°F (175°C) for 12 to 15 minutes or until thoroughly heated. Serve hot.

Yield:	12 servings
Exchange:	(1 serving) 1/2 medium-fat meat, 1/3 bread
Calories:	(1 serving) 63
Carbohydrates:	(1 serving) 5 grams

BACON-RINGED EGGS

1	bacon slice	1
1	egg	1
1/2 cup	mashed potatoes	125 milliliters
	salt & pepper to taste	
	fresh parsley for garnish	

A nice Sunday brunch dish for the family or just for a single serving. Lightly oil the bottom of a custard cup. Curl the bacon slice around the inside of the cup. (If you prefer the bacon crisp, fry slightly before lining the cup.) Break the egg inside the bacon ring. Season with salt and pepper to taste. Bake at 350°F (175°C) for about 15 to 20 minutes or until egg is firm but not hard. (Cooking time will vary with the number of bacon-egg dishes you are baking.) Carefully remove egg and bacon together from the cup to avoid separating bacon from egg. Place in the middle of the mashed potatoes. Garnish with parsley. Serve hot.

Yield:	1 serving
Exchange:	(1 serving) 1 bread, 1 1/2 medium-fat meat
Calories:	(1 serving) 188
Carbohydrates:	(1 serving) 15 grams

EGGS BAKED IN SHELLS

1/4 **cup**	low-calorie margarine (melted)	60 milliliters
1/4 **cup**	all-purpose flour	60 milliliters
1/2 **teaspoon**	salt	2 milliliters
1/8 **teaspoon**	black pepper	1/2 milliliter
2 cups	skim milk	500 milliliters
1/2 **cup**	sharp Cheddar cheese	125 milliliters
6	eggs	6

This is a lovely dish to serve. Combine the margarine, flour, salt, pepper, and milk in a saucepan; stir to thoroughly blend. Cook and stir until mixture just starts to thicken. Stir in the cheese; cook until cheese melts. Divide evenly among 6 shell baking dishes; allow to cool slightly to thicken. With the back of a spoon, make a hollow or indentation in the cheese sauce and break 1 egg in each. Season with salt and pepper. Place filled shells on a baking sheet. Cover lightly with aluminum foil. Bake at 350°F (175°C) for 15 to 20 minutes or until eggs are firm but not hard.

       Yield: 6 servings
 Exchange: (1 serving) 1 1/2 medium-fat meat, 3/4 bread,
               1/2 low-fat milk
   Calories: (1 serving) 235
Carbohydrates: (1 serving) 16 grams

COTTAGE EGGS

3	asparagus spears	3
1	egg	1
1 ounce	Swiss cheese (grated)	30 grams
	salt & pepper to taste	

Steam asparagus spears until tender. Place in individual baking dish. Poach egg; add salt and pepper. Place on top of asparagus. Top with cheese. Broil until cheese melts.

     Yield: 1 serving
 Exchange: 2 high-fat meat, 1 vegetable
  Calories: 216

EGGS WITH MORNAY SAUCE

2 tablespoons	low-calorie margarine	30 milliliters
2 tablespoons	all-purpose flour	30 milliliters
$^1/_2$ teaspoon	salt	2 milliliters
	pepper to taste (freshly ground)	
1	small bay leaf	1
$1^1/_2$ teaspoons	fresh parsley (minced)	7 milliliters
2 teaspoons	onion (minced)	10 milliliter
1 cup	skim milk	250 milliliters
2 tablespoons	Gruyère cheese	30 milliliters
6	eggs	6

Melt margarine in a saucepan. Add flour, salt, pepper, bay leaf, parsley, and onion; stir to blend. Slowly add the milk. Cook and stir until thickened; remove the bay leaf. Stir in the cheese; remove pan from heat. Arrange 6 custard cups on a baking pan. Pour 1 tablespoon (15 milliliters) of the sauce into each cup; break an egg over the sauce. Cover egg with an additional 2 tablespoons (30 milliliters) of the sauce. Bake at 350°F (175°C) for 15 to 20 minutes or until eggs are firm but not hard. Serve immediately.

Yield:	6 servings
Exchange:	(1 serving) $^1/_3$ bread, 1 high-fat meat
Calories:	(1 serving) 114
Carbohydrates:	(1 serving) 4 grams

MONTANA EGGS

1	egg (beaten)	1
$^1/_2$ ounce	ham (finely chopped)	15 grams
1 teaspoon	onion (finely chopped)	5 milliliters
	salt & pepper to taste	
	vegetable cooking spray	

Combine egg, ham, onion, salt, and pepper in small bowl. Beat to blend. Coat pan with vegetable cooking spray; heat to moderately hot. Add egg mixture. Cook on low heat; stir to scramble.

Yield:	1 serving
Exchange:	$1^1/_2$ high-fat meat
Calories:	125

MEATY EGG TART

Crust:	³/₄ cup	all-purpose flour	190 milliliters
	¹/₄ cup	vegetable shortening	60 milliliters
3¹/₂ tablespoons		ice water	52 milliliters
Filling:	1	bacon slice	1
	3	broccoli stalks (not florets)	3
	1	garlic clove	1
	5	mushrooms (sliced)	5
¹/₂ pound		ground beef	250 grams
	5	eggs (slightly beaten)	5
¹/₄ cup		skim milk	60 milliliters

Crust: Combine the flour and shortening in a bowl or food processor. Cut into pea-sized pieces. Fold in the ice water to make a dough. Chill for at least an hour. Roll into a thin crust. Place in bottom of 8-inch (20-centimeter) tart pan. Prick sides and bottom with fork. Bake at 425°F (220° C) for 15 minutes. Remove piecrust from oven.

Filling: Fry bacon in a skillet. Peel and slice broccoli stalks into thin slices. Remove bacon from skillet, crumble, and set aside. To remaining bacon fat in skillet, add the garlic, mushrooms, and broccoli. Sauté until mushrooms are limp. Remove vegetables and set aside. Add ground beef and cook over medium heat until meat loses its pink color; drain thoroughly. In a bowl, combine the crumbled bacon, vegetables, beef, eggs, and milk; stir to blend. Pour into piecrust. Bake at 425°F (220°C) for 15 minutes; reduce heat to 350°F (175°C) and bake 30 minutes longer or until completely set. Allow to rest 5 minutes before cutting.

Yield:	8 servings
Exchange:	(1 serving) 1 bread, 2 medium-fat meat, ¹/₂ fat
Calories:	(1 serving) 240
Carbohydrates:	(1 serving) 16 grams

BAKED POTATO WITH EGG

3	medium potatoes	3
3 tablespoons	skim milk	45 milliliters
	salt & pepper to taste	
6	eggs	6
	paprika	

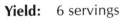

Wash and scrub the potatoes. Bake at 425°F (220°C) about 40 minutes or until tender. Reduce oven heat to 350°F (175°C). Cut potatoes lengthwise in half. Carefully scoop out potatoes in a small bowl without breaking the skins. Mash potatoes with the milk. (If potatoes seem dry, add a small amount of hot water.) Beat until light and fluffy. Fill potato skins, leaving a hollow in the middle. Break an egg in each hollow. Season with salt and pepper and sprinkle with paprika. Place back in oven and bake about 7 minutes until egg is firm but not hard.

> **Yield:** 6 servings
> **Exchange:** (1 serving) 1 medium-fat meat, ¹/₂ bread
> **Calories:** (1 serving) 115
> **Carbohydrates:** (1 serving) 8 grams

HERBED EGGS IN RAMEKINS

4	eggs (hard-cooked)	4
1 teaspoon each	basil, thyme, sweet marjoram, parsley	5 milliliters each
2 tablespoons	low-calorie margarine	30 milliliters
2	eggs (slightly beaten)	2
¹/₄ cup	skim evaporated milk	60 milliliters
¹/₄ cup	skim milk	60 milliliters
	salt & pepper to taste	

Melt margarine in a saucepan. Add the herbs and sauté for several minutes. Mince the hard-cooked eggs. Remove saucepan from heat and add remaining ingredients; stir to blend. Divide mixture evenly among 4 well-greased ramekins or custard cups. Place ramekins in a pan of hot water. Bake at 350°F (175°C) for 20 minutes or until firm.

> **Yield:** 4 servings
> **Exchange:** (1 serving) 2 medium-fat meat
> **Calories:** (1 serving) 160
> **Carbohydrates:** (1 serving) 2 grams

EGGS ON SPANISH RICE

2 cups	long-grain rice (cooked)	500 milliliters
6-ounce can	tomato paste	180-gram can
1 1/2 cups	water	375 milliliters
1/2 cup	onion (chopped)	125 milliliters
1/2 teaspoon	salt	2 milliliters
1	bay leaf	1
2	whole cloves	2
2 tablespoons	butter (melted)	30 milliliters
2 tablespoons	all-purpose flour	30 milliliters
6	eggs	6

Arrange rice in layer on bottom of well-greased baking dish. To make the Spanish sauce, combine tomato paste, water, onion, salt, bay leaf, and cloves in a saucepan. Cook and stir over medium heat for 10 minutes or until well blended and hot; remove bay leaf and cloves. Blend in the butter and flour; cook and stir until mixture is smooth and thickened. Make 6 hollows or indentations in the rice and break an egg into each indentation. Pour the sauce over eggs and rice. Bake at 350°F (175°C) for 15 to 20 minutes or until eggs are firm but not hard. Serve hot.

Yield: 6 servings
Exchange: (1 serving) 1 bread, 1 medium-fat meat
Calories: (1 serving) 148
Carbohydrates: (1 serving) 16 grams

POACHED EGGS WITH WINE

1 teaspoon	butter	5 milliliters
1/2 cup	Rhine wine	125 milliliters
4	eggs	4
	salt & pepper to taste	
2 tablespoons	Blue cheese (crumbled)	30 milliliters

Melt butter in a skillet. Add the wine. Carefully slip eggs into skillet. Season with salt and pepper. Cover and cook over medium heat until egg whites are set but egg is still loose. Sprinkle with the cheese. Cover and continue cooking until eggs are done as you like them and cheese is melted.

Yield: 4 servings
Exchange: (1 serving) 1 medium-fat meat, 1/2 bread
Calories: (1 serving) 114
Carbohydrates: (1 serving) 7 grams

EGGS FLORENTINE

3 cups	spinach (cooked)	750 milliliters
6	eggs	6
	salt & pepper to taste	
¹/₂ cup	sharp Cheddar cheese (grated)	125 milliliters
¹/₂ cup	skim evaporated milk	125 milliliters
¹/₂ cup	skim milk	125 milliliters
2 cups	bread crumbs (toasted)	500 milliliters

A must recipe for any breakfast or brunch cookbook. Place cooked spinach in bottom of shallow baking dish; make 6 hollows in the spinach. Drop an egg into each hollow and season with salt and pepper. To prepare the cheese sauce, mix the cheese, evaporated milk, and skim milk in the top of a double boiler over boiling water; heat until the cheese melts and the sauce thickens. Pour the hot sauce over the eggs and spinach. Sprinkle with bread crumbs. Bake at 350°F (175°C) for about 25 minutes until brown. Serve hot.

Yield: 6 servings
Exchange: (1 serving) 1 medium-fat meat, I vegetable, 2 bread
Calories: (1 serving) 235
Carbohydrates: (1 serving) 36 grams

OLD-FASHIONED POACHED EGG

2 cups	water	500 milliliters
1 teaspoon	white vinegar	5 milliliters
¹/₂ teaspoon	salt	2 milliliters
¹/₄ teaspoon	black pepper	1 milliliter
1	egg (slightly beaten)	1
1	bread slice (toasted)	1

Heat water to the boiling point in a small skillet. Add the vinegar, salt, and pepper. Break egg into a cup and gently slip into the boiling water. With a spoon or fork, make a whirlpool effect in the water. Reduce heat to allow water to simmer. Cook until egg is firm. Remove egg with a skimmer; drain and serve on toast.

Yield: 1 serving
Exchange: (1 serving) 1 medium-fat meat, 1 bread
Calories: (1 serving) 148
Carbohydrates: (1 serving) 14 grams

EGG-MUSHROOM CREAM SAUCE ON MUFFINS

4	eggs (hard-cooked)	4
1/2 cup	skim milk	125 milliliters
1/4 cup	evaporated skim milk	60 2milliliters
2 teaspoons	all-purpose flour	10 milliliters
1/2 cup	snow-capped mushrooms (sliced)	125 milliliters
1/4 pound	Cheddar cheese (grated)	125 grams
	salt & pepper to taste	
3	English muffins	3
	fresh parsley for garnish (optional)	

Slice or chop the eggs. Scald 1/4 cup (60 milliliters) milk and the evaporated milk in top of a double boiler. In a bowl, blend remaining milk and flour into a smooth paste. Stir flour mixture into the scalded milk. Add eggs, mushrooms, and cheese. Season with salt and pepper. Cook and stir over simmering water until cheese melts. Break muffins in half and toast. Place each half muffin on a heated plate. Evenly divide cream sauce among the 6 muffins. If desired, garnish with fresh parsley. Serve immediately.

Yield: 6 servings
Exchange: (1 serving) 1 bread, 1 high-fat meat, 1/2 fat
Calories: (1 serving) 198
Carbohydrates: (1 serving) 17 grams

EGGS DELUXE

4	bread slices (toasted)	4
4	eggs (separated)	4
	salt & pepper to taste	

Moisten edges of the toast with hot water. In a skillet, bring a small amount of salted water to the boiling point. Poach the egg yolks until soft-cooked. Place one egg yolk in middle of each piece of toast. Whip egg whites until stiff; spread or pipe with a pastry tube around the yolk. Season with salt and pepper. Bake at 350°F (175°C) for about 4 to 5 minutes until whites are slightly browned.

Yield: 4 servings
Exchange: (1 serving) 1 bread, 1 medium-fat meat
Calories: (1 serving) 148
Carbohydrates: (1 serving) 14 grams

DELIGHTFUL EGGS

1 cup	corned beef (chopped finely)	250 milliliters
1 cup	dry bread crumbs (finely crushed)	250 milliliters
¹/₃ cup	skim milk	90 milliliters
4 cups	mashed potatoes	1 liter
8	eggs (poached)	8
2	tomatoes (sliced)	2
8	green pepper rings	8

An easy way to deliver eggs and meat to the table and still have time for your guests. Mix the corned beef, bread crumbs, and milk in a bowl to make a paste. (If more moisture is needed, add small amounts of water to get the desired paste consistency.) Spread the meat-bread mixture on the bottom of a lightly greased tart pan; *do not* let mixture touch sides of pan. Place mashed potatoes in a pastry tube fitted with a large decorative opening. Pipe an edging around the meat-bread mixture. Divide the central circle of meat-bread mixture into 8 even triangles by piping the remaining mashed potatoes into a spoke design. Slip a poached egg into each triangle. Bake at 425°F (220°C) until potato is browned. Garnish with tomato slices and pepper slices. Serve immediately.

Yield:	8 servings
Exchange:	(1 serving) 1¹/₂ medium-fat meat, 1¹/₂ bread
Calories:	(1 serving) 251
Carbohydrates:	(1 serving) 21 grams

EGGS BENEDICT

half	English muffin	half
1 ounce	lean ham slice	30 grams
1	egg	1
1 tablespoon	Hollandaise sauce (page 164)	15 milliliters
	salt & pepper to taste	

Toast muffin half. Cook ham over low heat. Place on muffin. Poach egg and place on top of ham. Spoon Hollandaise Sauce over egg. Add salt and pepper.

Yield:	1 serving
Exchange:	2¹/₂ high-fat meat, ¹/₂ bread, 1 fat
Calories:	266

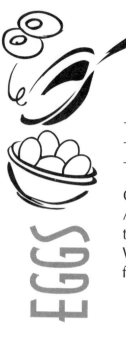

BASIC OMELET

1	egg (well beaten)	1
	salt & pepper to taste	
	vegetable cooking spray	

Coat pan with vegetable cooking spray; heat pan to moderately hot. Add beaten egg and cook over low heat. Lift edges of egg very carefully to allow uncooked portion of egg to run under. Add salt and pepper. When mixture is firm, fold omelet in half, or roll up jelly-roll style. A filling may be added before folding.

Yield: 1 serving
Exchange: 1 medium-fat meat
Calories: 78

MICROWAVE OMELET

3	eggs (separated)	3
¹/₂ cup	sour cream	125 milliliters
2 tablespoons	green onion (sliced)	30 milliliters
2 tablespoons	tomato flesh	30 milliliters
1 tablespoon	parsley (snipped)	15 milliliters
¹/₂ cup	ham (cooked & diced)	125 milliliters
	salt & pepper to taste	

Beat egg whites in a bowl until stiff; In another bowl, beat egg yolks until very thick and creamy; beat in the sour cream. Stir in the remaining ingredients. Season with salt and pepper to taste. Gently fold in the beaten egg whites. Place mixture in a 9- or 10-inch (23- or 25-centimeter) lightly greased pie pan; cover lightly with plastic wrap (make sure there is enough room for the eggs to expand). Cook in microwave on MEDIUM for 5 minutes, turning dish a half turn every minute. Allow to rest 1¹/₂ minutes before serving.

Yield: 6 servings
Exchange: (1 serving) 1 high-fat meat, 1 fat
Calories: (1 serving) 169
Carbohydrates: (1 serving) negligible

EGGS AND CHICKEN LIVERS

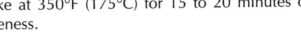

4	chicken livers	4
4	eggs	4
4 tablespoons	2 percent milk	60 milliliters
	salt & freshly ground pepper to taste	
	paprika	

Place chicken livers in a small skillet. Add a small amount of water and simmer until livers are thoroughly cooked; drain. Cut livers into small pieces. Divide among 4 well-oiled ramekins, baking shells, or custard cups; break an egg over the liver pieces in each ramekin. Add 1 tablespoon (15 milliliters) milk to each cup; sprinkle with salt, pepper, and paprika. Bake at 350°F (175°C) for 15 to 20 minutes or until set to desired doneness.

Yield:	4 servings
Exchange:	(1 serving) 1½ medium-fat meat
Calories:	(1 serving) 120
Carbohydrates:	(1 serving) negligible

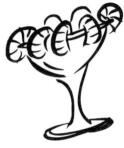

SHRIMP DIP

5 small	shrimp	5 small
1/2 teaspoon	Worcestershire sauce	2 milliliters
1 teaspoon	lemon juice	5 milliliters
4 ounces	plain lo-cal yogurt	120 grams
1/4 cup	Chili Sauce (page 166)	60 milliliters

Crush shrimp. Sprinkle with Worcestershire sauce and lemon juice. Combine yogurt and Chili Sauce. Add crushed shrimp; stir to blend. Chill.

> **Yield:** 3/4 cup (190 milliliters)
> **Exchange:** 1 meat, 1/2 milk, 1/2 fruit
> **Calories:** 108

CHEESE APPETIZERS

4 ounces	Cheddar cheese (shredded)	120 grams
2 tablespoons	margarine	30 milliliters
1/2 cup	flour	125 milliliters
1 teaspoon	onion (grated)	5 milliliters
1/2 teaspoon	salt	2 milliliters
1/4 teaspoon	pepper	1 milliliter

Blend cheese and margarine until smooth. Add flour, onion, salt, and pepper. Stir until smooth. Shape dough into a roll, 1 1/4 inches (3.5 centimeters) in diameter. Wrap in plastic wrap or aluminum foil. Chill. Cut into 1/4-inch (6 millimeter) slices. Bake at 400°F (200°C) for 8 minutes.

> **Yield:** 24 servings
> **Exchange:** (1 serving) 1/2 fat, 1/4 bread
> **Calories:** (1 serving) 37

STUFFED CELERY

2	5-inch (12$\frac{1}{2}$-centimeter) celery stalks	2
1 tablespoon	cream cheese (softened)	15 milliliters
$\frac{1}{4}$ teaspoon	onion powder	1 milliliter
dash	paprika	dash
	salt & pepper to taste	

Thoroughly rinse and drain celery. Combine cream cheese, onion powder, and paprika. Blend until smooth and creamy. Add salt and pepper. Fill celery stalks. Chill.

Yield: 1 serving
Exchange: 1 fat
Calories: 50

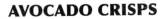

AVOCADO CRISPS

1	very ripe avocado	1
1 teaspoon	lemon juice	5 milliliters
1 teaspoon	grated onion	5 milliliters
1 teaspoon	onion salt	5 milliliters
1 teaspoon	paprika	5 milliliters
$\frac{1}{2}$ teaspoon	marjoram	2 milliliters
	thin crackers	

Peel and mash avocado. Add remaining ingredients. Beat until smooth. Spread thinly on crackers.

Yield: 45 servings
Exchange: (5 servings) 1 bread, 1 fat
Calories: (5 servings) 108

APPETIZERS

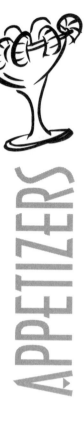

CUCUMBERS IN YOGURT

1	cucumber	1
1 small	onion	1 small
1 teaspoon	salt	5 milliliters
1/2 teaspoon	garlic powder	2 milliliters
1 teaspoon	lemon juice	5 milliliters
1/2 teaspoon	marjoram	2 milliliters
8 ounces	lo-cal yogurt	240 grams

Peel and thinly slice cucumber and onion. Sprinkle with salt. Allow to rest 15 minutes. Drain and pat dry. Combine garlic powder, lemon juice, marjoram, and yogurt; mix thoroughly. Fold in sliced cucumber and onion. Chill.

Yield: 2 cups (500 milliliters)
Exchange: 1 milk
Calories: 100

SUMMER CHICKEN CANAPÉS

4 ounces	ground cooked chicken	120 grams
2 tablespoons	margarine (softened)	30 milliliters
1/4 teaspoon	dry mustard	1 milliliter
1/2 teaspoon	meat tenderizer	2 milliliters
1/2 teaspoon	salt	2 milliliters
1/8 teaspoon	pepper	1/2 milliliter
1/4 inch thick	cucumber slices	6 millimeters thick

Combine chicken, margarine, dry mustard, meat tenderizer, salt, and pepper. Mix thoroughly. Chill. To make canapé: Place 1 teaspoon (5 milliliters) of chicken mixture in center of cucumber slice.

Yield: 24 servings
Exchange: (2 servings) 1/2 fat
Calories: (2 servings) 28

GARLIC BITES

1 slice	white bread	1 slice
2 teaspoons	lo-cal margarine	10 milliliters
¹/₄ teaspoon	garlic pwder	1 milliliter

Remove crust from bread; cut bread into ¹/₄-inch (6 millimeter) cubes. Melt margarine in small pan. Add garlic powder and heat until sizzling. Add bread cubes; sauté, tossing frequently until brown. Drain and cool.

Yield: 2 servings
Exchange: (1 serving) ¹/₂ bread, 1 fat
Calories: (1 serving) 79

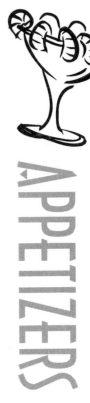

LIVER PASTE

3 ounces	chicken livers	90 grams
1 tablespoon	onion (finely chopped)	15 milliliters
1	egg (hard cooked)	1
2 teaspoons	margarine	10 milliliters
1 tablespoon	evaporated (regular or skim) milk	15 milliliters
	salt & pepper to taste	

Boil chicken livers and onion in small amount of water until tender. Drain. Finely chop the egg. Mash livers, onion, egg, and margarine until well blended. Add milk; blend thoroughly. Add salt and pepper.

Yield: 24 servings, 1 teaspoon (5 millimeters) each
Exchange: (3 servings) ¹/₂ medium-fat meat
Calories: (3 servings) 39

SWISS MORSELS

8 ounces	Swiss cheese (grated)	240 grams
4 ounces	ham (grated)	120 grams
2 tablespoons	margarine (softened)	30 milliliters
¹/₄ teaspoon	thyme	1 milliliter

Combine all ingedients; mix thoroughly. Shape 2 teaspoons (10 milliliters) of mixture into a ball. Repeat with remaining mixture.

Yield: 34 servings
Exchange: (1 serving) ¹/₂ high-fat meat
Calories: (1 serving) 51

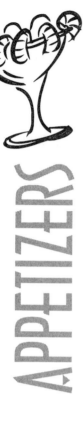

SMOKED SALMON CANAPÉS

8 ounces	smoked salmon	240 grams
3 ounces	cream cheese	90 grams
1/2 teaspoon	lemon juice	2 milliliters
1 teaspoon	milk	5 milliliters
dash each	thyme, sage, salt, pepper	dash each

Place smoked salmon in blender. Blend until fine. Combine cream cheese, lemon juice, and milk. Stir to make a paste. Add seasonings. Mix well. Add salmon; blend thoroughly. Roll into 22 balls. Chill.

      Yield: 22 servings
Exchange: (2 servings) 1 meat
  Calories: (2 servings) 68

HORS D'OEUVRE SPREADS

      Yield: 1/4 cup (60 milliliters) spread for 24 crackers or
                1/2 teaspoon (2 milliliters) per cracker
Exchange: (per serving) 1/2 fat plus cracker exchange

Use one of the following as a spread for 24 small crackers:

ANCHOVY

1 ounce	anchovy fillets	30 grams
1/4 cup	lo-cal margarine	60 milliliters

Rinse fillets in cold water; pat dry. Grind or chop fine; blend with margarine. Allow to rest.

Exchange: (1/4 cup/60 milliliters) 12 fat, 1 meat
 Calories: (1/4 cup/60 milliliters) 250

CAVIAR

2 tablespoons	caviar	30 milliliters
1/4 cup	lo-cal margarine	60 milliliters

Combine caviar and margarine. Refrigerate overnight.

Exchange: (1/4 cup/60 milliliters) 12 fat, 1 meat
 Calories: (1/4 cup/60 milliliters) 280

APPETIZERS

CRABMEAT

2 tablespoons	crabmeat	30 milliliters
¹/₄ cup	lo-cal margarine	60 milliliters

Crush crabmeat; blend with margarine. Refrigerate overnight.

Exchange: (¹/₄ cup/60 milliliters) 12 fat, ¹/₂ meat
Calories: (¹/₄ cup/60 milliliters) 230

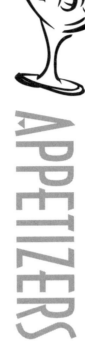

GARLIC

¹/₄ teaspoon	garlic	1 milliliter
dash	salt	salt
¹/₄ cup	lo-cal margarine	60 milliliters

Blend ingredients together.

Exchange: (¹/₄ cup/60 milliliters) 12 fat
Calories: (¹/₄ cup/60 milliliters) 200

HERB

dash each	onion (chopped), marjoram, oregano, salt, pepper	dash each
¹/₄ cup	lo-cal margarine	60 milliliters

Blend ingredients together; allow to rest at room temperature 2 hours.

Exchange: (¹/₄ cup/60 milliliters) 12 fat
Calories: (¹/₄ cup/60 milliliters) 200

HORSERADISH

1 tablespoon	horseradish (grated)	15 milliliters
1 teaspoon	parsley (chopped)	5 milliliters
¹/₄ cup	lo-cal margarine	60 milliliters

Blend ingredients together; refrigerate overnight.

Exchange: (¹/₄ cup/60 milliliters) 12 fat
Calories: (¹/₄ cup/60 milliliters) 200

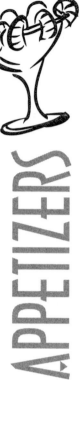

LEMON

1 teaspoon	lemon juice	5 milliliters
dash	salt	dash
¹/₄ teaspoon	parsley	1 milliliter
¹/₄ cup	lo-cal margarine	60 milliliters

Blend ingredients together.

Exchange: (¹/₄ cup/60 milliliters) 12 fat
Calories: (¹/₄ cup/60 milliliters) 200

MUSTARD

2 teaspoons	Dijon mustard	10 milliliters
¹/₄ cup	margarine	60 milliliters

Blend ingredients together.

Exchange: (¹/₄ cup/60 milliliters) 12 fat
Calories: (¹/₄ cup/60 milliliters) 200

Note: Exchange and calorie figures above do not include crackers.

Spreads may be topped with:

1 teaspoon	chicken, chicken liver, ham, salami, sausage, tuna, crabmeat, or lobster	5 milliliters
Exchange: **to add 6 crackers**	1 meat (plus cracker exchange)	
1 teaspoon	bacon, avocado	5 milliliters
Exchange: **to add 5 crackers**	1 fat (plus cracker exchange)	
1 teaspoon	cauliflower, celery, cucumber, mushroom, onion, parsley, radish, green pepper, or tomato flesh	5 milliliters
Exchange:	only cracker exchange	

SALADE NICOISE

¹/₂ cup	Dia-Mel red wine vinegar salad dressing	125 milliliters
¹/₂ cup	Dia-Mel Italian salad dressing	125 milliliters
¹/₂ teaspoon	dried dill	2 milliliters
¹/₂ teaspoon	oregano	2 milliliters
dash	black pepper	dash
¹/₂	red or yellow onion (thinly sliced)	¹/₂
3 ounces	marinated artichoke hearts (drained)	90 grams
1 cup	fresh green beans (cut & trimmed) or frozen French-style green beans (thawed & drained)	250 milliliters
2 small	Boston lettuce (torn into bite-size pieces)	2
¹/₂	cucumber (sliced)	¹/₂
2	tomatoes (cut in wedges)	2
¹/₂ cup	mushrooms (sliced)	125 milliliters
¹/₄ cup	radishes (sliced)	60 milliliters
¹/₂ cup	red pepper (sliced in thin strips)	125 milliliters
1 medium	potato (cooked & sliced)	1 medium
7-ounce can	tuna (packed in water, rinsed)	200-gram can
¹/₄ cup	pitted black olives (sliced)	60 milliliters
1	egg (hard-cooked & chopped)	1

Combine salad dressing with dill, oregano and pepper. Marinate onion, artichoke hearts and green beans in dressing mixture for 2 to 3 hours. Before serving, combine the marinated vegetables and dressing with the remaining ingredients *except* the hard-cooked egg. Toss to mix well. Garnish with the chopped egg.

Yield: 4 servings
Exchange: (1 serving) 2 lean meat, 3 vegetables
Calories: (1 serving) 180

For you from The Estee Corporation.

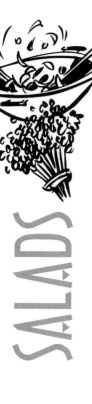

MUSHROOM & WATERCRESS SALAD

3 cups	snow-white mushrooms (medium size)	750 milliliters
2 tablespoons	fresh lemon juice	30 milliliters
2 tablespoons	white wine vinegar	30 milliliters
2 tablespoons	olive oil	30 milliliters
1/3 cup	water	90 milliliters
1/2 teaspoon	salt	2 milliliters
1/2 teaspoon	dried tarragon (crushed)	2 milliliters
1/4 teaspoon	ground basil	1 milliliter
1 cup	fresh watercress (chopped)	250 milliliters

Clean and slice mushrooms; place in a medium bowl. Mix together the lemon juice, vinegar, oil, water, salt, tarragon and basil. Pour dressing over mushrooms, mixing carefully to completely coat the mushrooms. Marinate overnight in the refrigerator. Just before serving, drain extra dressing from mushrooms, add watercress and toss to completely mix. Divide among 8 chilled salad plates.

Yield: 8 servings
Exchange: (1 serving) 1/2 vegetable, 1 fat
Calories: (1 serving) 57

APPLE-CABBAGE SLAW

1/4 cup	Dia-Mel creamy Italian salad dressing	60 milliliters
1/4 teaspoon	prepared mustard	1 milliliter
dash	pepper	dash
2 cups	cabbage (shredded)	500 milliliters
1 cup	unpared apple (thinly sliced)	250 milliliters

In a medium bowl, combine salad dressing, mustard and pepper. Add cabbage and apple and toss lightly. Serve immediately.

Yield: 4 servings
Exchange: (1 serving) 1 1/2 vegetable
Calories: (1 serving) 35

For you from The Estee Corporation.

POINSETTIA SALAD

1 cup	Stone-Buhr brown rice (cooked)	250 millilitres
7-ounce can	chunk-style tuna (drained)	200-gram can
¹/₂ cup	pecans (chopped)	125 millilitres
¹/₃ cup	mayonnaise	90 millilitres
1 tablespoon	lemon juice	15 millilitres
¹/₄ teaspoon	Tabasco sauce	1 millilitre
1	canned whole pimiento	1
6	lettuce leaves	6

Cook rice according to package directions. Rinse with cold water and drain well. Combine tuna, rice, pecans, mayonnaise, lemon juice and Tabasco sauce. Toss lightly until well mixed. Press into 6 individual moulds or use a ¹/₃-cup (90 millimetres) measure. Turn out each moulded salad onto a lettuce leaf. Cut pimiento into petal shapes and arrange on salads to resemble poinsettias.

Yield: 6 servings
Exchange: (1 serving) 2 bread, 1 high-fat meat, 2 fat
Calories: (1 serving) 335

With the compliments of Arnold Foods Company, Inc.

VEGETABLE-BEAN SALAD

8-ounce can	Featherweight cut green beans (drained)	227-gram can
8-ounce can	Featherweight cut wax beans (drained)	227-gram can
¹/₂ cup	green or red pepper (chopped)	125 milliliters
¹/₄ cup	onion (sliced)	60 milliliters
¹/₂ cup	Featherweight Italian dressing	125 milliliters
6	lettuce leaves	6

In a medium bowl, combine all ingredients except the lettuce. Cover and marinate overnight in the refrigerator. Serve on lettuce.

Yield: 6 servings
Exchange: (1 serving) 1 vegetable
Calories: (1 serving) 31

Based on a recipe from Featherweight Brand Foods.

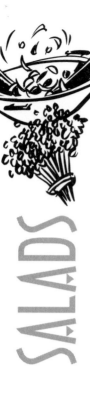

SALADS

POLYNESIAN CABBAGE SLAW

1 small	cabbage (shredded)	1 small
8¹/₂-ounce can	pineapple chunks packed in juice	230-gram can
1	orange (diced)	1
¹/₄ cup	green pepper (diced)	60 milliliters
¹/₃ cup	Dia-Mel Thousand Island salad dressing	90 milliliters
¹/₃ cup	Dia-Mel French-style salad dressing	90 milliliters
¹/₃ cup	Dia-Mel catsup	90 milliliters

Drain pineapple chunks. In a large bowl, combine all ingredients and mix thoroughly. Chill before serving.

Yield:	6 servings
Exchange:	(1 serving) 1 fruit, ¹/₂ vegetable
Calories:	(1 serving) 55

For you from The Estee Corporation.

OLD-TIME CARROT SLAW

¹/₃ cup	water	90 milliliters
2 tablespoons	vegetable oil	30 milliliters
2 tablespoons	white vinegar	30 milliliters
3 packets	aspartame sweetener	3 packets
¹/₂ teaspoon	salt	2 milliliters
dash	black pepper	dash
3 cups	carrots (shredded)	750 milliliters
8	ripe olives (sliced)	8

Combine water, oil, vinegar, aspartame, salt and pepper. Stir to blend. Pour over carrots. Toss to completely coat. Garnish with olive slices. Cover tightly and chill thoroughly. Drain well before serving.

Yield:	6 servings
Exchange:	(1 serving) 1 vegetable, 1 fat
Calories:	(1 serving) 73

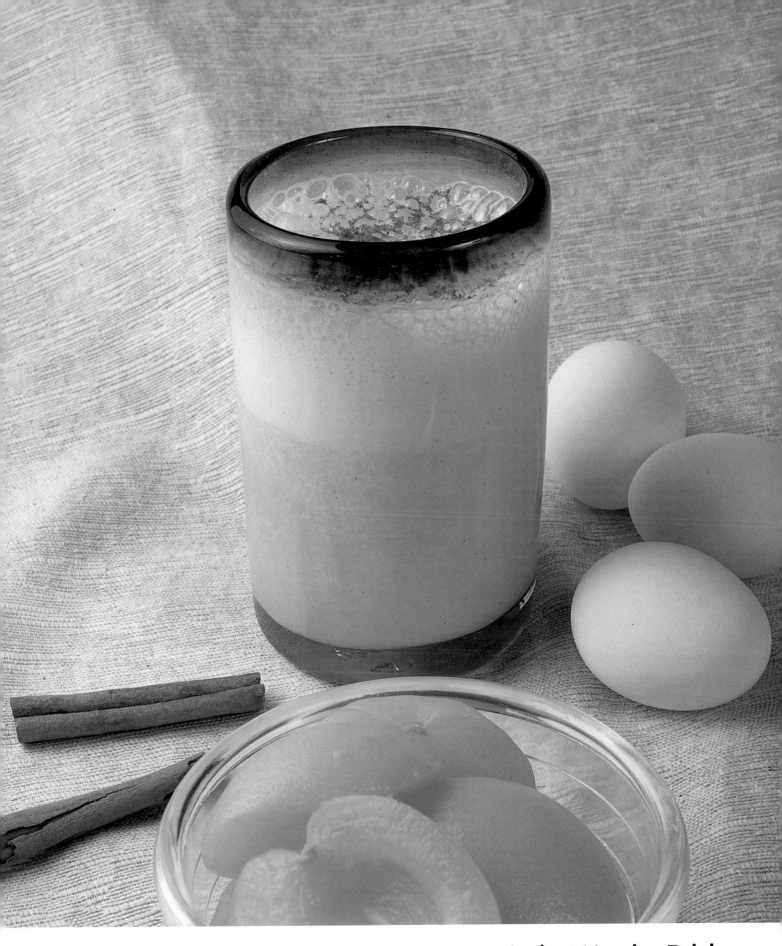

Apricot Morning Drink

• • •

see page 12

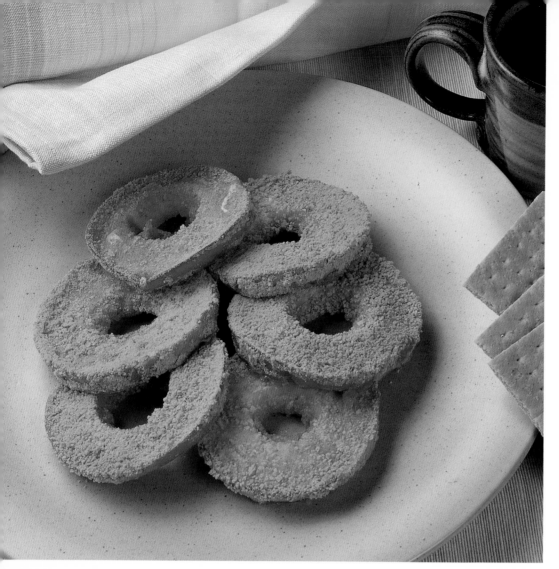

Baked Apples

•••

see page 15

Sunshine Stollen

•••

see page 26

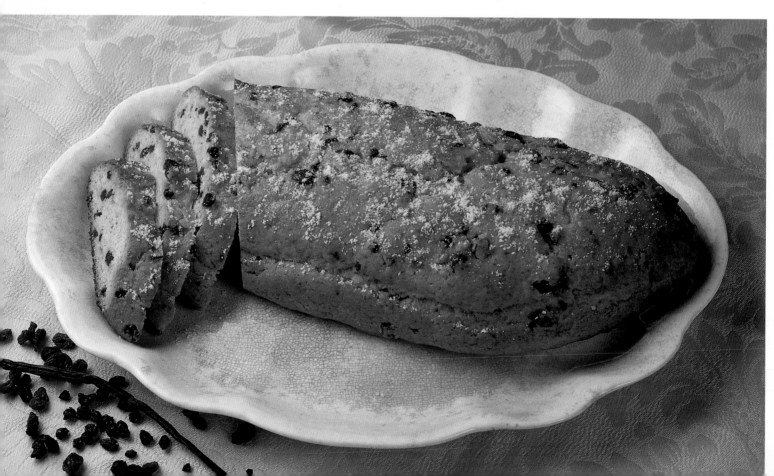

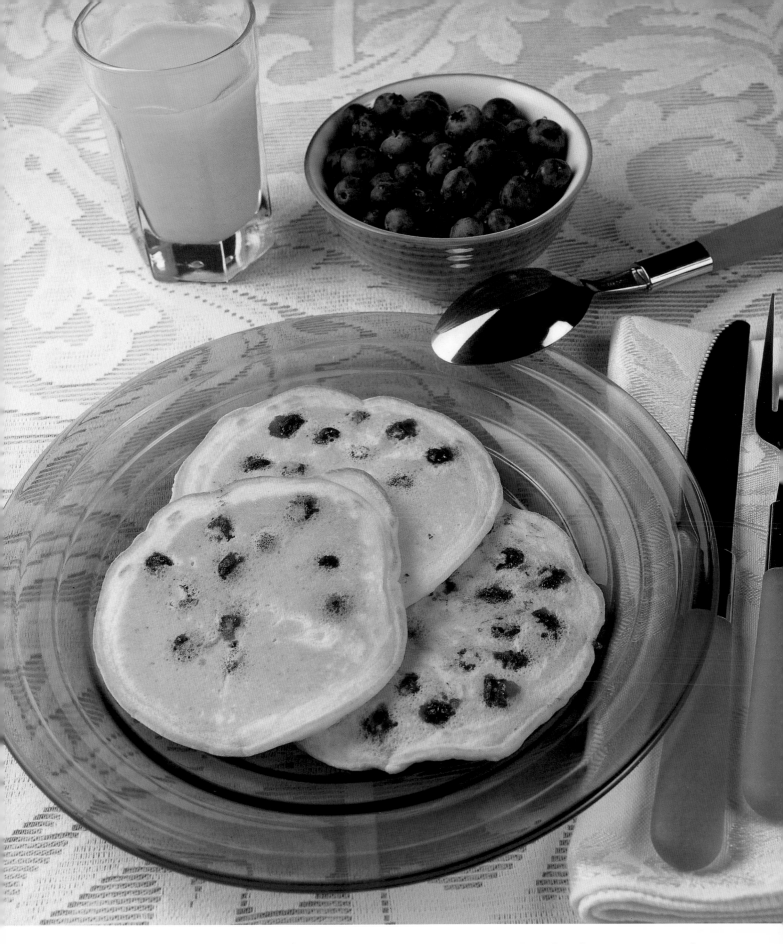

Fresh Blueberry Pancakes

• • •

see page 23

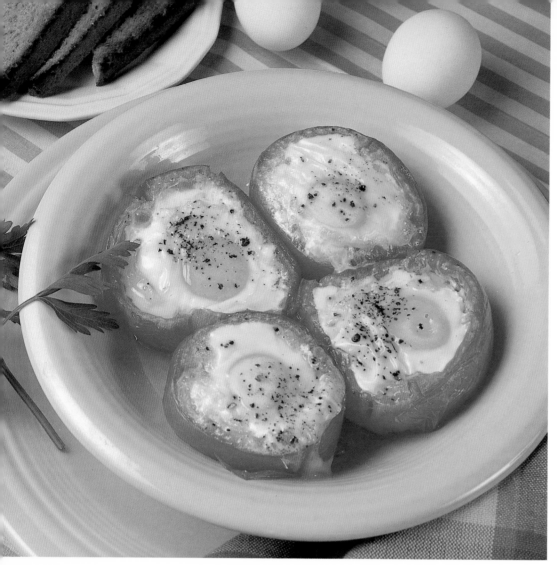

Eggs in Tomato Nests

• • •

see page 42

Avocado Crisps

• • •

see page 55

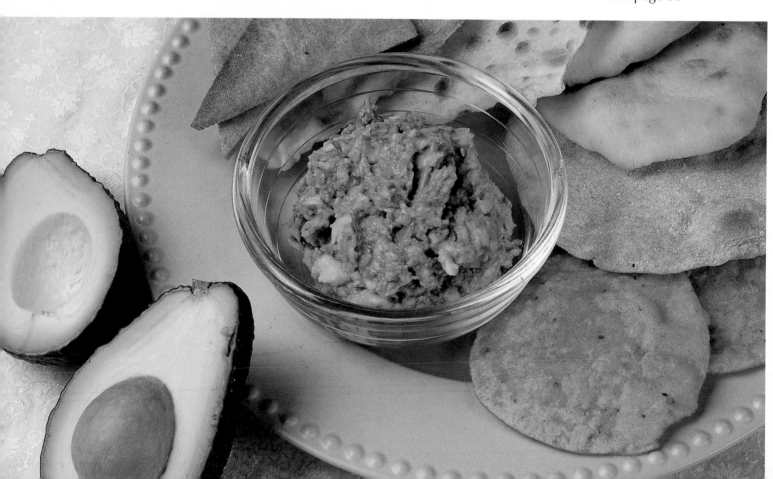

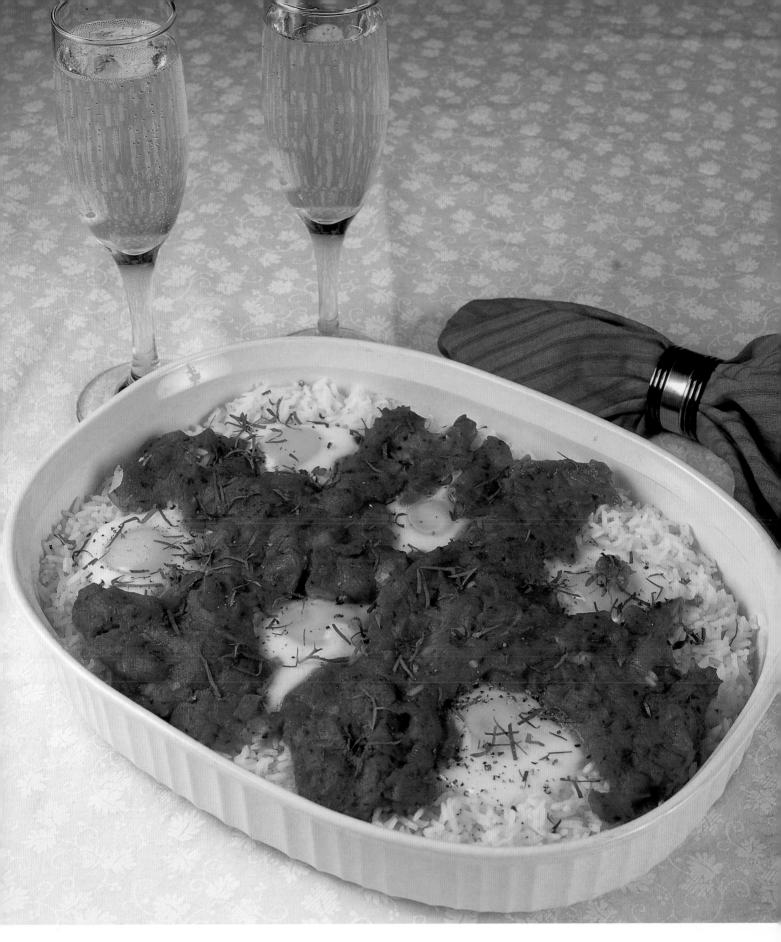

Eggs on Spanish Rice
• • •
see page 48

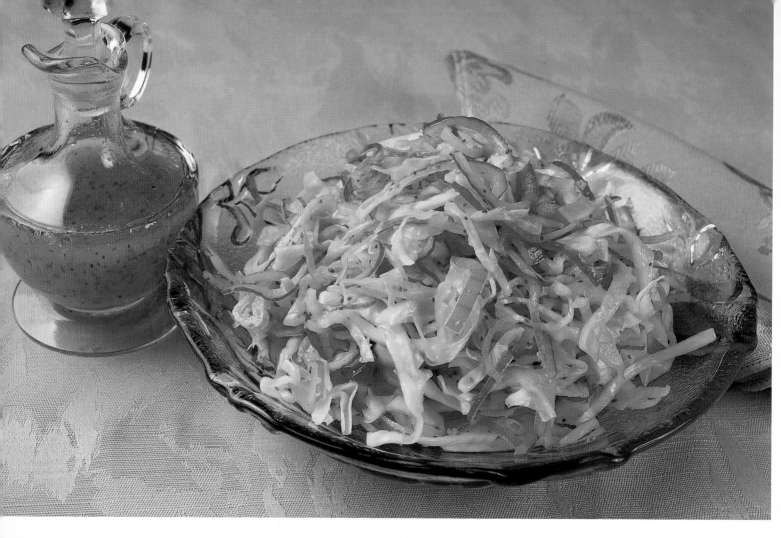

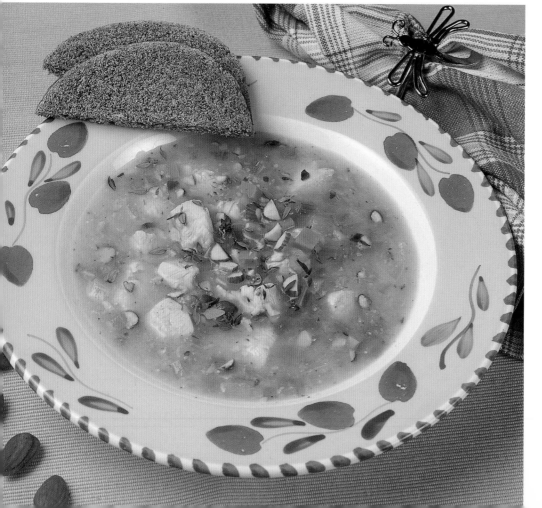

Sweet-Sour Slaw

• • •

see page 65

Cream of Chicken & Almond Soup

• • •

see page 75

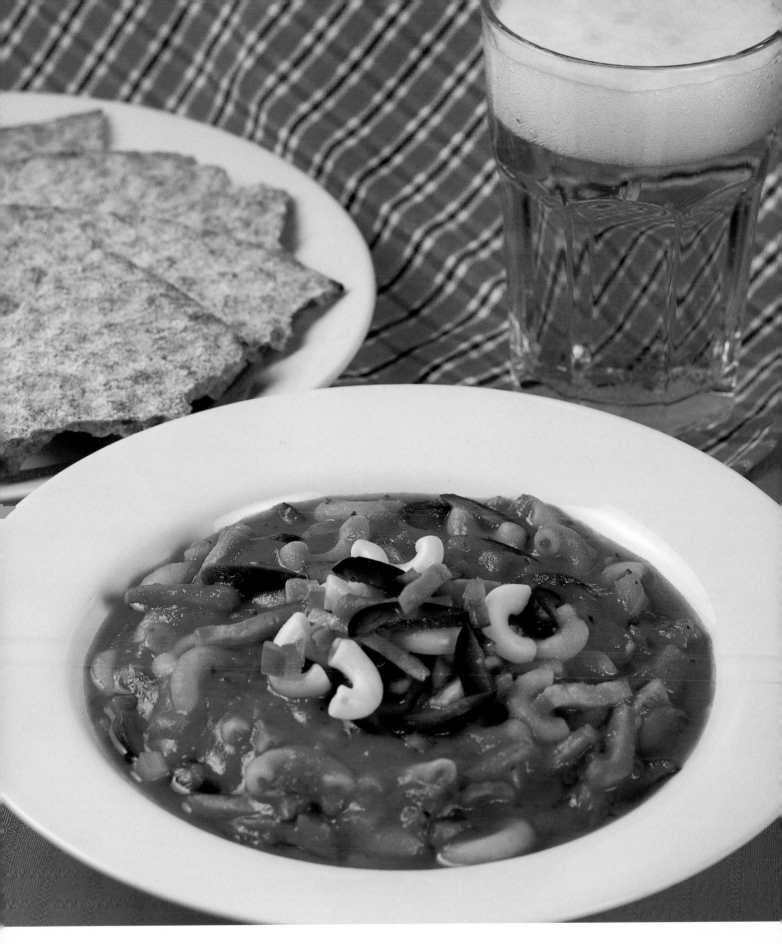

Pizza Stew

• • •

see page 78

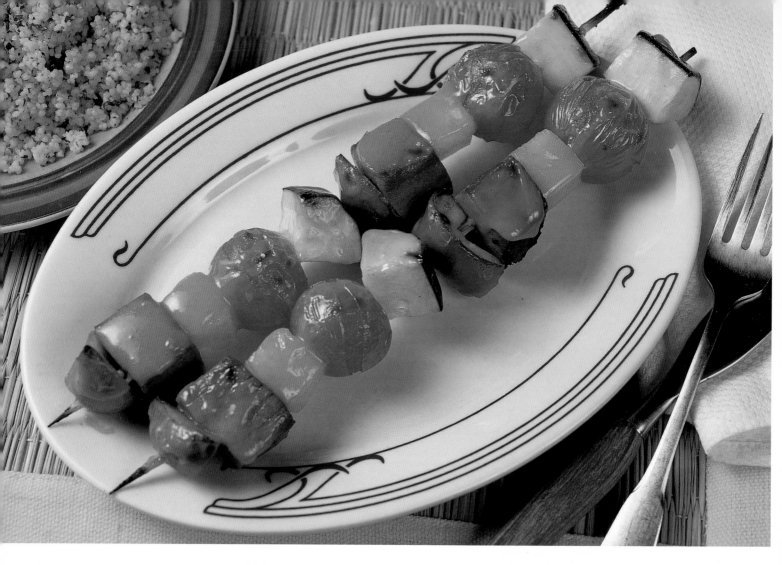

Quick Kabobs

• • •

see page 84

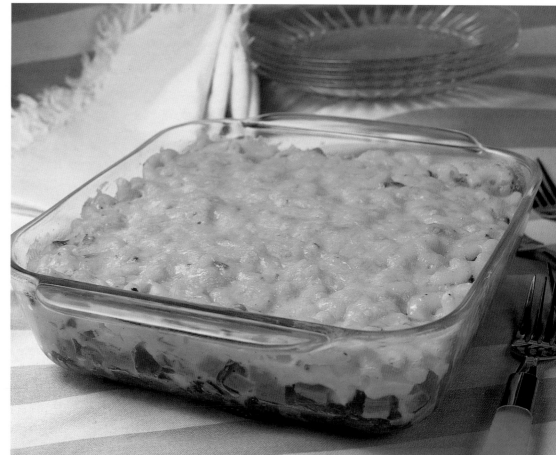

Macaroni & Cheese Supreme

• • •

see page 89

SWEET-SOUR SLAW

2 medium	red onions	2 medium
4 cups	cabbage (finely shredded)	1 liter
¹/₂ cup	cider vinegar	125 milliliters
1 teaspoon	dry mustard	5 milliliters
1 teaspoon	salt	5 milliliters
1 teaspoon	celery seeds	5 milliliters
¹/₄ teaspoon	cornstarch	1 milliliter
¹/₃ cup	granulated sugar replacement	90 milliliters
2 tablespoons	vegetable oil	30 milliliters

Thinly slice the onions and separate them into rings. In a large bowl, alternate layers of the cabbage and onion rings. In a small saucepan, combine vinegar, mustard, salt, celery seeds and cornstarch. Stir to dissolve cornstarch. Cook over medium heat until mixture boils and is clear. Remove from heat, beat in sugar replacement and oil. Pour dressing over the cabbage. Cover tightly and refrigerate 8 hours or overnight, stirring occasionally. To serve, using a slotted spoon, lift salad out of the dressing.

Yield: 10 servings
Exchange: (1 serving) ¹/₂ fat
Calories: (1 serving) 25

LEMONY APPLE-BRAN SALAD

¹/₂ cup	lemon low-fat yogurt	125 milliliters
1 tablespoon	fresh parsley (finely snipped)	15 milliliters
2 cups	unpared red apples (cored & cubed)	500 milliliters
¹/₂ cup	celery (thinly sliced)	125 milliliters
¹/₂ cup	red grapes (halved & seeded)	125 milliliters
¹/₂ cup	All-Bran or Bran Buds cereal	125 milliliters
6	lettuce leaves	6

Stir together yogurt, parsley, apples, celery and grapes. Cover and chill thoroughly. At serving time, stir in the cereal. Serve on lettuce leaves.

Yield: 6 servings
Exchange: (1 serving) 1 fruit, ¹/₂ bread
Calories: (1 serving) 70

From Kellogg's Test Kitchens.

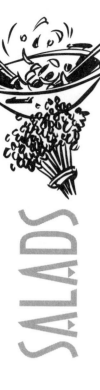

HOT BEAN SALAD

2 cups	kidney beans (cooked & drained)	500 milliliters
1 cup	celery (thinly sliced)	250 milliliters
$^1/_2$ cup	sharp American cheese (diced)	125 milliliters
$^1/_4$ cup	sweet relish	60 milliliters
$^1/_4$ cup	onions (coarsely chopped)	60 milliliters
$^1/_3$ cup	low-cal mayonnaise	90 milliliters
$^1/_2$ teaspoon	salt	2 milliliters
$^1/_3$ cup	wheat germ	90 milliliters

Combine beans, celery, cheese, relish, onions, mayonnaise, and salt in a large bowl. Stir to mix thoroughly. Spoon into 8 custard cups or baking dishes. Sprinkle wheat germ on top. Bake at 450°F (230°C) for 10 minutes or until bubbly.

Yield: 8 servings
Exchange: (1 serving) $^2/_3$ bread, 1 lean meat
Calories: (1 serving) 97

CHILLED BEAN SALAD

15$^1/_2$-ounce can	no-salt-added green beans	450-gram can
15$^1/_2$-ounce can	no-salt-added wax beans	450-gram can
1	red pepper (chopped)	1
12	cherry tomatoes (cut in half)	12
$^1/_2$ teaspoon	dried dill	2 milliliters
$^1/_2$ teaspoon	dried basil	2 milliliters
$^1/_4$ cup	Dia-Mel red wine vinegar salad dressing	60 milliliters

Drain green and wax beans and combine with the red pepper and tomatoes. Add dillweed and basil to salad dressing; stir to combine. Pour dressing over vegetables and toss gently. Chill for several hours or overnight.

Yield: 6 servings
Exchange: (1 serving) 1$^1/_2$ vegetable
Calories: (1 serving) 40

For you from The Estee Corporation.

WILTED LETTUCE SALAD

2 tablespoons	margarine	30 milliliters
³/₄ teaspoon	paprika	3 milliliters
¹/₄ teaspoon	garlic salt	1 milliliter
1 tablespoon	sesame seeds	15 milliliters
1 cup	All-Bran or Bran buds cereal	250 milliliters
2 tablespoons	Parmesan cheese (grated)	30 milliliters
6	bacon slices	6
2 quarts	iceberg lettuce (torn into bite-size pieces)	2 liters
1	tomato (chopped)	1
¹/₄ cup	green onions (sliced)	60 milliliters
¹/₂ teaspoon	oregano	2 milliliters
¹/₄ teaspoon	pepper	1 milliliter
¹/₄ cup	vinegar	60 milliliters
2 teaspoons	sugar	10 milliliters

In a medium skillet, melt margarine over low heat. Stir in paprika, garlic salt and sesame seeds. Add cereal, stirring until well-coated. Cook, stirring constantly, 2 to 3 minutes or until cereal is crisp and lightly brown. Remove from heat. Add cheese, tossing lightly. Set aside.

Fry bacon until crisp. Drain, reserving 2 tablespoons (30 milliliters) of the drippings. Crumble bacon into small pieces. Set aside. In a large bowl, toss lettuce with tomato, green onions, oregano and pepper. Set aside. Combine reserved bacon drippings, vinegar and sugar in a small saucepan. Bring to a boil. Pour over lettuce. Cover bowl about 1 minute. Portion salad into individual salad bowls. Sprinkle bacon and cereal mixture over each portion. Serve immediately.

Yield: 6 servings
Exchange: (1 serving) ¹/₂ bread, 2 vegetables, 2 fat
Calories: (1 serving) 175

From Kellogg's Test Kitchens.

67

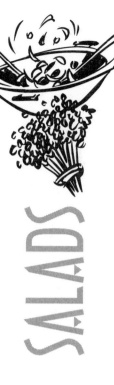

SALADS

MINTED BROWN RICE SALAD

2¹/₂ cups	brown rice (cooked & hot)	625 milliliters
¹/₃ cup	lemon juice	90 milliliters
2 tablespoons	vegetable oil	30 milliliters
¹/₂ cup	fresh parsley (minced)	125 milliliters
¹/₂ cup	fresh mint (minced)	125 milliliters
¹/₄ cup	green onions (thinly sliced)	60 milliliters
¹/₂ cup	dates (finely chopped)	125 milliliters
¹/₂ teaspoon	salt	2 milliliters
2	oranges	2

Combine hot rice, lemon juice, oil, parsley, mint, onions, dates and salt in large bowl. Stir to completely blend. Cover and refrigerate until thoroughly chilled. Mound rice in a chilled, shallow serving dish. Peel oranges; slice crosswise. Decorate rice salad with the orange slices.

Yield: 6 servings
Exchange: (1 serving) 1 bread, 1 fruit, 1 fat
Calories: (1 serving) 155

TABBOULEH

¹/₂ cup	Stone-Buhr cracked wheat	125 milliliters
3 medium	fresh tomatoes (finely chopped)	3 medium
1 cup	parsley (finely chopped)	250 milliliters
1 cup	onion (finely chopped)	250 milliliters
¹/₃ cup	fresh lemon juice	90 milliliters
2 teaspoons	salt	10 milliliters
1 tablespoon	vegetable oil	15 milliliters

Soak cracked wheat in cold water for about 10 minutes; drain. Wrap in cheesecloth and squeeze until dry. In large bowl, combine cracked wheat, tomatoes, parsley, onion, lemon juice and salt; toss lightly with a fork. Marinate at least half hour before serving. Just before serving, stir in oil.

Yield: 8 servings
Exchange: (1 serving) ²/₃ bread, ¹/₂ fat
Calories: (1 serving) 63

With the compliments of Arnold Foods Company, Inc.

CHICKEN BROTH

2-pound	hen (cut up)	1-kilogram
¹/₂ medium	stalk celery (chopped)	¹/₂ medium
8 to 10	green onions (chopped)	8 to 10
2 tablespoons	parsley (chopped)	30 milliliters
2 teaspoons	salt	10 milliliters
1 teaspoon	thyme	5 milliliters
1 teaspoon	marjoram	5 milliliters
¹/₂ teaspoon	pepper	2 milliliters

Wash chicken pieces; place in large kettle. Cover with 2 quarts (2 liters) water; bring to boil, cover and cook 1 hour or until chicken is tender. Add remaining ingredients; simmer 1 hour. Remove chicken; strain broth. Refrigerate broth overnight. Remove all fat from surface before reheating broth.

Yield: 2 quarts (2 liters) broth
Exchange: Negligible
Calories: Negligible

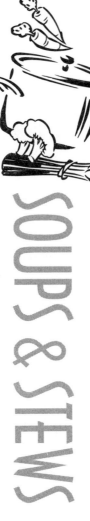

BEEF BROTH

3 to 4 pounds	beef soup bones or chuck roast	1¹/₂ to 2 kilograms
¹/₂ stalk	celery (chopped)	¹/₂ stalk
3	carrots (sliced)	3
1 medium	onion (chopped)	1 medium
¹/₂	green pepper (chopped)	¹/₂
2	bay leaves	2
¹/₂ teaspoon each	thyme, marjoram, paprika, pepper	2 milliliters each
2 teaspoons	salt	10 milliliters

Place beef in large kettle; cover with 2 quarts (2 liters) water. Bring to a boil, cover and cook 2 hours, or until meat is tender. Add remaining ingredients; simmer 1 hour. Remove beef; strain broth. Refrigerate broth overnight. Remove all fat from surface before reheating broth.

Yield: 2 quarts (2 liters) broth
Exchange: Negligible
Calories: Negligible

SOUPS & STEWS

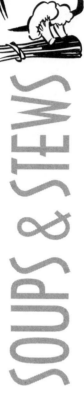

VEGETABLE BROTH

1 cup	onion (chopped)	250 milliliters
2 cups	carrots (diced)	500 milliliters
1 cup	celery (chopped)	250 milliliters
2 cups	spinach (cut in small pieces)	500 milliliters
2 cups	tomato (peeled & chopped)	500 milliliters
1	bay leaf	1
2 tablespoons	parsley or parsley flakes	30 milliliters
1/2 teaspoon	thyme	2 milliliters
1 blade	mace	1 blade
1/4 teaspoon	garlic or garlic powder	1 milliliter
1 tablespoon	Worcestershire sauce	15 milliliters
	salt to taste	

Place vegetables in large kettle. Cover with 2 to 3 quarts (2 to 3 liters) water. Bring to boil; reduce heat and simmer for 2 hours. Stir frequently. Add seasonings. Simmer 1 hour. Strain. Add water to make 2 quarts (2 liters).

Yield: 2 quarts (2 liters) broth
Exchange: Negligible
Calories: Negligible

BROTH ITALIANO

1/8 cup	vermicelli (broken)	30 milliliters
1 cup	broth	250 milliliters
1 ounce	thinly sliced prosciutto (shredded)	30 grams
1/8 teaspoon	garlic powder	1/2 milliliter
1/8 teaspoon	marjoram	1/2 milliliter
1 tablespoon	Parmesan cheese (grated)	15 milliliters

Cook vermicelli in boiling salted water; drain and rinse. Bring broth to boil. Add prosciutto, garlic powder, and marjoram. Simmer 5 minutes. Add vermicelli. Pour into bowl. Sprinkle Parmesan cheese over top.

Yield: 1 1/4 cups (310 milliliters)
Exchange: 1/2 bread, 1 medium-fat meat
Calories: 107

BROTH ORIENTALE

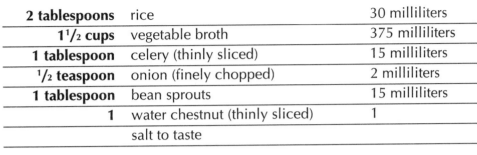

2 tablespoons	rice	30 milliliters
1¹/₂ cups	vegetable broth	375 milliliters
1 tablespoon	celery (thinly sliced)	15 milliliters
¹/₂ teaspoon	onion (finely chopped)	2 milliliters
1 tablespoon	bean sprouts	15 milliliters
1	water chestnut (thinly sliced)	1
	salt to taste	

Add rice to cold vegetable broth; bring to a boil. Reduce heat; simmer 20 minutes. Add celery, onion, bean sprouts and water chestnut; simmer 10 minutes. Add salt.

Microwave: Add rice to cold broth; heat to a boil. Cover. Hold 15 minutes. Add remaining ingredients, except salt. Cook 3 minutes. Hold 5 minutes. Add salt.

> **Yield:** 1¹/₄ cups (310 milliliters)
> **Exchange:** ¹/₈ bread, ¹/₈ vegetable
> **Calories:** 11

BROTH WITH VEGETABLES

Cook ¹/₂ cup (125 milliliters) vegetables or combination of vegetables in boiling salted water; drain. Add to hot broth just before serving.

Microwave: Add ¹/₂ cup (125 milliliters) vegetables (no water needed). Cook on HIGH for 3 minutes. Add to hot broth just before serving.

> **Yield:** ¹/₂ cup (125 milliliters)
> **Exchange:** ¹/₂ vegetable
> **Calories:** 18

BROTH WITH NOODLES

Cook ¹/₄ cup (60 milliliters) noodles or broken spaghetti in boiling salted water; drain. Add to hot broth just before serving.

Microwave: Add ¹/₄ cup (60 milliliters) noodles or pasta to 2 cups (500 milliliters) boiling salted water. Cook on HIGH for 3 minutes. Hold 3 minutes. Drain. Add to hot broth just before serving.

> **Yield:** ¹/₂ cup (125 milliliters)
> **Exchange:** 1 bread
> **Calories:** 68

SOUPS & STEWS

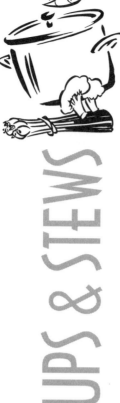

BROTH MADEIRA

Add 1 tablespoon (15 milliliters) Madeira to 1 cup (250 milliliters) broth. Bring just to a boil. Garnish with lemon slice and fresh chopped parsley.

Microwave: Add 1 tablespoon (15 milliliters) Madeira to 1 cup (250 milliliters) broth. Cook on HIGH for 2 minutes. Garnish with lemon slice and fresh chopped parsley.

Yield:	1 cup (250 milliliters)
Exchange:	Negligible
Calories:	Negligible

GREEK EGG LEMON SOUP

2 quarts	chicken broth	2 litres
3	eggs (separated)	3
	juice of 1 lemon	

Bring broth to a boil in saucepan. Beat egg whites until stiff. Add egg yolks. Beat slowly until mixture is a light yellow. Add lemon juice gradually, beating constantly. Pour small amount of chicken broth into egg mixture. Pour egg mixture into hot broth, beating constantly.

Yield:	8 servings, 1 cup (250 milliliters) each
Exchange:	(1 serving) ¼ high-fat meat
Calories:	(1 serving) 27

QUICK EGG SOUP

1½ cups	boiling water	375 milliliters
1 cube	vegetable bouillon	1 cube
1	egg	1

Dissolve bouillon cube in boiling water; remove from heat. Beat egg; blend into vegetable broth. Reheat slowly. DO NOT BOIL.

Yield:	1½ cups (375 milliliters)
Exchange:	1 medium-fat meat
Calories:	80

BORSCH

16-ounce can	beets with juice	500-gram can
2 tablespoons	sugar replacement	30 milliliters
³/₄ teaspoon	salt	3 milliliters
3 tablespoons	lemon juice	45 milliliters
¹/₂ teaspoon	thyme	2 milliliters
1	egg (well beaten)	1

Puree beets in blender. Add enough water to make 1 quart (1 liter). Pour into saucepan. Add sugar replacement, salt, lemon juice, and thyme; heat to a boil. Remove from heat. Add small amount of hot beet mixture to egg. Stir egg mixture into beet mixture. Return to heat; cook and stir until hot.

Added touch: Top each serving with 1 teaspoon (5 milliliters) lo-cal sour cream.

> **Yield:** 4 servings, 1 cup (250 milliliters) each
> **Exchange:** (1 serving) 1 bread, ¹/₄ high-fat meat
> **Calories:** (1 serving) 104

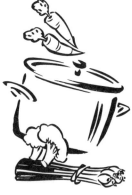

GERMAN CABBAGE SOUP

2 ounces	ground beef round	60 grams
2 tablespoons	onion (grated)	30 milliliters
dash each	mustard, soy sauce, salt, pepper	dash each
1 tablespoon	dry red wine	15 milliliters
1¹/₄ cups	beef broth	310 milliliters
2 large	cabbage leaves (cut in pieces)	2 large
¹/₂ medium	tomato (cubed)	¹/₂ medium
¹/₂ teaspoon	fresh parsley (chopped)	2 milliliters

Combine ground round, onion, mustard, soy sauce, salt, and pepper; mix thoroughly. Form into tiny meatballs. Add wine to broth; bring to boil. Add meatballs to broth, one at a time. Bring to boil again. Cook meatballs 5 minutes; remove to soup bowl. Add cabbage and tomatoes to broth. Simmer 5 minutes. Pour over meatballs. Garnish with parsley.

> **Yield:** 1¹/₂ cups (375 milliliters)
> **Exchange:** 1 medium-fat meat, ¹/₂ vegetable
> **Calories:** 55

SOUPS & STEWS

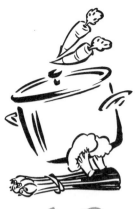

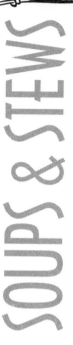

TOMATO BEEF BOUILLON

2 tablespoons	margarine	30 milliliters
¼ cup	onion (chopped)	60 milliliters
46 ounces	tomato juice	1½ liters
2 cans	beef broth **or**	2 cans
2½ cups	homemade beef broth	625 milliliters
1	bay leaf	1
1 teaspoon	salt	5 milliliters
½ teaspoon	pepper	2 milliliters

Heat margarine in large saucepan. Add onion and cook until tender. Add tomato juice, beef broth (canned or homemade), bay leaf, salt, and pepper; heat thoroughly.

DO NOT BOIL. Remove bay leaf. Ladle into warm bowls.

Added Touch: Top each serving with 1 teaspoon (5 milliliters) grated American cheese.

Yield: 8 servings, 1 cup (250 milliliters) each
Exchange: (1 serving) ¼ vegetable, 1 fat
Calories: (1 serving) 58

HAM AND SPLIT PEA SOUP

2 pounds	meaty ham bone	1 kilogram
1	bay leaf	1
2 cups	dried green split peas	500 milliliters
1 cup	onions (chopped)	250 milliliters
1 cup	celery (cubed)	250 milliliters
1 cup	carrots (grated)	250 milliliters
	salt & pepper to taste	

Cover ham bone and bay leaf with water. Simmer for 2 to 2½ hours. Remove bone and strain liquid. Refrigerate overnight. Remove lean meat from bone; set aside. Remove fat from surface of liquid. Heat liquid; add enough water to make 2½ quarts (2½ liters). Add peas; simmer for 20 minutes. Remove from heat and allow to stand 1 hour. Add onions, celery, carrots, and lean pieces of ham. Add salt and pepper. Simmer for 40 minutes. Stir occasionally.

Yield: 10 servings
Exchange: (1 serving) ½ high-fat meat, 1 vegetable
Calories: (1 serving) 204

CREAM OF CHICKEN & ALMOND SOUP

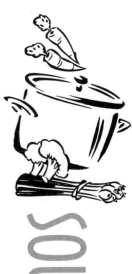

1 cup	chicken broth	250 milliliters
1	whole clove	1
1 sprig	parsley	1 sprig
¹/₂	bay leaf	¹/₂
pinch	mace	pinch
1 tablespoon	celery (sliced)	15 milliliters
1 tablespoon	carrot (diced)	15 milliliters
1 teaspoon	onion (diced)	5 milliliters
2 teaspoons	stale bread crumbs	10 milliliters
¹/₂ ounce	chicken breast (cubed)	15 grams
1 teaspoon	blanched almonds (crushed)	5 milliliters
¹/₄ cup	skim milk	60 milliliters
1 teaspoon	flour	5 milliliters
	salt & pepper to taste	

Heat chicken broth, clove, parsley, bay leaf, and mace to a boil; remove from heat. Allow to rest 10 minutes; strain. Add celery, carrot, onion, bread crumbs, chicken and almonds to seasoned chicken broth; simmer 20 minutes. Blend in skim milk and flour. Remove soup from heat; add milk mixture. Return to heat. Simmer (DO NOT BOIL) 3 to 5 minutes. Add salt and pepper.

Yield: 1¹/₂ cups (375 milliliters)
Exchange: ¹/₂ lean meat, 1 vegetable, ¹/₄ milk
Calories: 89

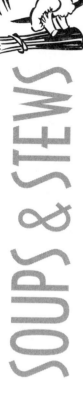

SOUPS & STEWS

FRENCH MEATBALL SOUP

2 tablespoons	rice (uncooked)	30 milliliters
2 ounces	ground beef round	60 grams
1 tablespoon	egg (raw, beaten)	15 milliliters
1 teaspoon	onion (grated)	5 milliliters
dash each	garlic, parsley, nutmeg	dash each
2 tablespoons	dry red wine	30 milliliters
1¼ cups	beef broth	310 milliliters
	salt & pepper to taste	

Add rice to 1 cup (250 milliliters) salted water. Boil 5 minutes; drain well. Blend rice, ground round, egg, onion, garlic, parsley, and nutmeg; form into small meatballs. Add wine to broth; bring to a boil. Drop meatballs into hot broth, one at a time. Bring to a boil again; reduce heat. Simmer 20 minutes. Add salt and pepper.

Microwave: Add rice to 1 cup (250 milliliters) salted water. Bring to a boil. Hold 5 minutes; drain well. Combine meatball ingredients as above. Bring wine and broth to a boil. Drop meatballs into hot broth, one at a time. Bring to a boil again. Hold 10 minutes. Add salt and pepper.

Yield: 1½ cups (375 milliliters)
Exchange: 1 medium-fat meat, ½ bread
Calories: 71

CRAB CHOWDER

1 cup	milk	250 milliliters
1 teaspoon	flour	5 milliliters
¼ cup	water	60 milliliters
¼ cup	cooked crabmeat (flaked)	60 milliliters
3 tablespoons	mushroom pieces	45 milliliters
3 tablespoons	asparagus pieces	45 milliliters
	salt & pepper to taste	

Blend milk, flour, and water thoroughly; pour into saucepan. Add crabmeat, mushrooms, and asparagus. Cook over low heat until slightly thickened. Add salt and pepper.

Yield: 1 cup (250 milliliters)
Exchange: 1 milk, 1 vegetable, 1 lean meat
Calories: 150

CLAM CHOWDER

1 slice	bacon	1 slice
1¹/₂ cups	fish or vegetable broth	375 milliliters
2 tablespoons	carrot (diced)	30 milliliters
1 tablespoon	onion (diced)	15 milliliters
1 tablespoon	celery (diced)	15 milliliters
1 large	tomato (diced)	1 large
1 medium	potato (diced)	1 medium
dash each	thyme, rosemary, salt, pepper	dash each
1 teaspoon	flour	5 milliliters
¹/₄ cup	water	60 milliliters
1 ounce	clams	30 grams

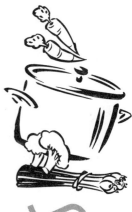

SOUPS & STEWS

Cook bacon until crisp; drain and crumble. Combine broth, carrot, onion, celery, tomato, potato, and seasonings. Simmer until vegetables are tender. Blend flour and water; stir into chowder. Reduce heat. Add clams and crumbled bacon. Heat to thicken slightly.

Microwave: Combine vegetables with broth and seasonings; cover. Cook on HIGH for 4 minutes, or until vegetables are tender. Add flour-water mixture. Cook 30 seconds; stir. Add clams and bacon; stir. Cook 30 seconds. Hold 3 minutes.

Yield: 2 cups (500 milliliters)
Exchange: 1 lean meat, 1 fat, 1 vegetable, 1 bread
Calories: 200

FISH CHOWDER

2 cups	water	500 milliliters
3 ounces	bullhead fillet	90 grams
1 medium	potato (diced)	1 medium
3 tablespoons	onion (diced)	45 milliliters
3 tablespoons	celery (diced)	45 milliliters
2 tablespoons	carrot (diced)	30 milliliters
1 medium	tomato (diced)	1 medium
	salt & pepper to taste	

Combine all ingredients in saucepan. Heat to a boil; cover and reduce heat. Simmer 1 to 1¹/₂ hours.

Yield: 3 servings, 1 cup (250 milliliters) each
Exchange: (1 serving) 1 medium-fat meat, ¹/₂ vegetable, ¹/₂ bread
Calories: (1 serving) 81

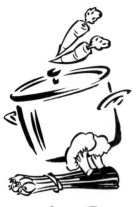

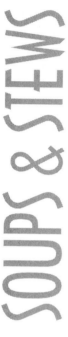

OYSTER STEW

1 teaspoon	flour	5 milliliters
1 tablespoon	celery (minced)	15 milliliters
1 teaspoon	salt	5 milliliters
dash each	Worcestershire sauce, soy sauce	dash each
1 tablespoon	water	15 milliliters
1 ounce	oysters (with liquid)	30 grams
1 teaspoon	butter	5 milliliters
1 cup	skim milk	250 milliliters

Blend flour, celery, seasonings, and water in saucepan; add oysters with liquid, and butter. Simmer over low heat until edges of oysters curl. Remove from heat; add skim milk. Reheat over low heat. Add extra salt if desired.

Yield: 1½ cups (375 milliliters)
Exchange: 1 lean meat, 1 milk, ¼ bread
Calories: 220

PIZZA STEW

1 ounce	Canadian bacon	30 grams
1½ cups	Tomato Sauce (page 168)	375 milliliters
¼ cup	water	60 milliliters
2 tablespoons	onion (chopped)	30 milliliters
1 tablespoon	mushroom pieces	15 milliliters
1 tablespoon	black olives (pitted & chopped)	15 milliliters
1 tablespoon	celery (chopped)	15 milliliters
1 tablespoon	green pepper (chopped)	15 milliliters
dash each	oregano, garlic powder, salt to taste	dash each
½ cup	elbow macaroni (cooked)	125 milliliters

Fry Canadian bacon; drain and cut away any fat. Heat Tomato Sauce and water to a boil. Add bacon, vegetables, and seasonings. Cook until vegetables are tender. Add macaroni; reheat.

Yield: 2¼ cups (560 milliliters)
Exchange: 1 high-fat meat, 1 bread, 1 vegetable
Calories: 275

KIDNEY STEW

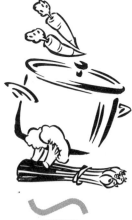

2 ounces	beef kidney (cooked)	60 grams
1½ cups	beef broth	375 milliliters
3 tablespoons	leek (chopped)	45 milliliters
1 slice	bacon (cooked & drained)	1 slice
¼ cup	mushrooms	60 milliliters
3 tablespoons	green pepper (sliced)	45 milliliters
dash each	parsley, thyme, tarragon, salt, pepper	dash each

Heat all ingredients to a boil. Reduce heat and simmer until green pepper slices are tender.

Yield:	1½ cups, (375 milliliters)
Exchange:	2 lean meat, 1 fat
Calories:	130

ZUCCHINI MEATBALL STEW

1 ounce	ground beef	30 grams
½ cup	ground zucchini	125 milliliters
1 teaspoon	onion (finely chopped)	5 milliliters
1	egg	1
¼ cup	rice (uncooked)	60 milliliters
dash each	oregano, cumin, garlic salt, pepper	dash each
1 cup	beef broth	250 milliliters
1 large	tomato (diced)	1 large
1 teaspoon	parsley (chopped)	5 milliliters
	salt & pepper to taste	

Combine ground beef, zucchini, onion, egg, rice, and seasonings; mix thoroughly. Shape into small meatballs. Combine beef broth, tomato, and parsley in saucepan; heat to boil. Drop meatballs into hot broth, one at a time. Cover and simmer 30 to 40 minutes. Add salt and pepper.

Microwave: Cook beef broth, tomato, and parsley on HIGH for 3 minutes, covered. Drop meatballs into broth. Cook on HIGH 5 minutes. Hold 10 minutes. Add salt and pepper.

Yield:	1¾ cups (430 milliliters)
Exchange:	2 medium-fat meat, 1 vegetable, 1 bread
Calories:	203

SOUPS & STEWS

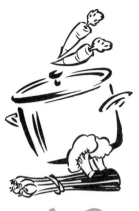

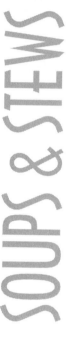

Soups & Stews

STEFADO

1 stick	cinnamon	1 stick
1	bay leaf	1
5	whole cloves	5
12 ounces	beef roast (cubed)	360 grams
	salt & pepper to taste	
1 teaspoon	margarine	5 milliliters
1½ cups	onions (sliced)	375 milliliters
3 medium	tomatoes (peeled & cubed)	3 medium
½ cup	red wine	125 milliliters
1 teaspoon	brown sugar replacement	5 milliliters
2 tablespoons	raisins	30 milliliters
1 cup	water	250 milliliters
1	garlic clove (crushed)	1

Place cinnamon, bay leaf, and cloves in small cheesecloth bag. Combine with remaining ingredients in soup kettle; cook 1 to 1½ hours until meat is tender. Remove spice bag before serving.

Microwave: Same as above. Cook on HIGH 15 to 20 minutes.

Yield: 3 servings, 1 cup (250 milliliters) each
Exchange: (1 serving) 4 high-fat meat, 1 vegetable
Calories: (1 serving) 430

PEPPER POT
(Leftovers may be used)

2 ounces	lean pork, cut in 1-inch (2.5-centimeter) cubes	60 grams
1 ounce	beef, cut in 1-inch (2.5-centimeter) cubes	30 grams
1 ounce	chicken, cut in 1-inch (2.5-centimeter) cubes	30 grams
¼ cup	carrot pieces	60 milliliters
¼ cup	onion slices	60 milliliters
¼ cup	celery pieces	60 milliliters
¼ cup	potatoes (cubed)	60 milliliters
½ cup	water	125 milliliters
1 teaspoon	flour	5 milliliters
dash each	curry powder, garlic powder, salt, pepper	dash each

Brown pork and beef cubes slowly in frying pan. Add chicken cubes for last few minutes; drain. Place meat, carrots, onions, celery, and potatoes in individual baking dish. Combine water, flour, and seasonings in screwtop jar; shake to blend well. Pour over meat mixture. Cover tightly and bake at 350°F (175°C) for 45 minutes to 1 hour, or until meat is tender and gravy has thickened.

Microwave: Reduce water to ¼ cup (60 milliliters). Cook on HIGH for 10 minutes. Hold 5 minutes.

Yield:	1 serving	
Exchange:	4 high-fat meat, 1 vegetable, 1 bread	
Calories:	418	

BEAN STEW

1 tablespoon	pinto beans	15 milliliters
1 tablespoon	northern beans	15 milliliters
1 tablespoon	lentils	15 milliliters
1 cup	beef broth	250 milliliters
1 tablespoon	carrot (sliced)	15 milliliters
1 tablespoon	hominy	15 milliliters
1 teaspoon	onion (diced)	5 milliliters
½ teaspoon	green chilies (chopped)	2 milliliters
dash each	garlic powder, oregano, salt, pepper	dash each

Boil beans and lentils in beef broth for 10 minutes, covered. Allow to stand 1 to 2 hours, or overnight. Place softened beans and remaining ingredients in baking dish. Bake at 350°F (175°C) for 45 minutes to 1 hour, or until ingredients are tender.

Microwave: Place beans and lentils in beef broth; cover. Cook on HIGH for 5 minutes. Allow to stand 1 to 2 hours or overnight. Add remaining ingredients. Cook on MEDIUM for 10 to 15 minutes, or until ingredients are tender.

Yield:	1½ cups, (375 milliliters)
Exchange:	1 lean meat, 2 bread
Calories:	225

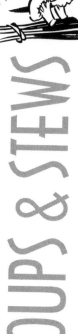

SOUPS & STEWS

CHICKEN GIBLET STEW

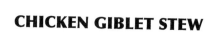

3 ounces	chicken giblets	90 grams
2 cups	water	500 milliliters
¼ teaspoon	thyme	1 milliliter
¼	bay leaf	¼
⅛ teaspoon	parsley (crushed)	½ milliliter
	salt & pepper to taste	
3 tablespoons	potatoes (diced)	45 milliliters
2 tablespoons	onions (diced)	30 milliliters
2 tablespoons	celery (diced)	30 milliliters
2 tablespoons	green beans (sliced)	30 milliliters
2 tablespoons	carrots (diced)	30 milliliters
2 tablespoons	peas	30 milliliters
1 teaspoon	flour	5 milliliters
¼ cup	water	60 milliliters

Remove center muscle of giblets. Place the 2 cups water, giblets, and seasonings in saucepan; cover. Heat to a boil; reduce heat and simmer until giblets are tender, about 1 hour. Add extra water to make about 2 cups (500 milliliters) liquid. Remove bay leaf. Add vegetables; reheat and cook until vegetables are tender. Blend flour with the ¼ cup water. Blend into stew. Cook to desired thickness.

Yield: 3 servings, 1 cup (250 milliliters) each
Exchange: (1 serving) 1 lean meat, 1 bread, 1 vegetable
Calories: (1 serving) 120

BEEF STROGANOFF

3 ounces	lean beef (cubed)	90 grams
1 teaspoon	margarine	5 milliliters
1/2	onion (cut into large pieces)	1/2
1/4 teaspoon	garlic (minced)	1 milliliter
2 tablespoons	mushroom pieces	30 milliliters
1/2 cup	condensed cream of mushroom soup	125 milliliters
1 tablespoon	lo-cal sour cream	15 milliliters
1 teaspoon	ketchup	5 milliliters
dash each	Worcestershire sauce, ground bay leaf, salt, pepper	dash each
1 cup	noodles	250 milliliters

Brown beef cubes in margarine. Add onion, garlic, and mushrooms. Cook over low heat until onion is partially cooked; remove from heat. Combine condensed soup, sour cream, ketchup, and seasonings; blend well. Pour over beef mixture; heat thoroughly (DO NOT BOIL). Serve over noodles.

Yield: 1 serving
Exchange: 3 high-fat meat, 2 1/2 bread
Calories: 470

PACKAGED STEAK SUPPER

3 ounces	beef minute steak	90 grams
1 small	potato	1 small
2 tablespoons	carrot (sliced)	30 milliliters
2 tablespoons	onion (sliced)	30 milliliters
2 tablespoons	celery (sliced)	30 milliliters
2 large	tomato slices	2 large
	salt & pepper to taste	

Place steak on large piece of aluminum foil. Layer vegetables in order given. Add salt and pepper. Wrap in foil, sealing ends securely. Bake at 350°F (175°C) for 1 hour.

Microwave: Place in plastic wrap. Cook on HIGH for 10 minutes.

Yield: 1 serving
Exchange: 3 medium-fat meat, 1 bread, 1/2 vegetable
Calories: 375

CASSEROLES & ONE-DISH MEALS

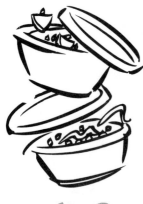

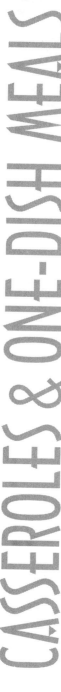

QUICK KABOBS

2 ounces	cooked roast beef, cut in 1-inch (2.5-centimeter) cubes	60 grams
6	green peppers, cut in 1-inch (2.5-centimeter) squares	6
6	cherry tomatoes	6
6	zucchini, cut in 1-inch (2.5-centimeter) cubes	6
6	unsweetened pineapple chunks	6
2 tablespoons	lo-cal French dressing	30 milliliters

Alternate beef, vegetables, and fruit on 2 skewers. Brush with 1 tablespoon (15 millilitres) of the French dressing. Broil 5 to 6 inches (12 to 15 centimeters) from heat for 8 minutes. Brush with remaining French dressing. Broil 4 minutes longer.

> **Yield:** 1 serving (2 kabobs)
> **Exchange:** 2 medium-fat meat, 1 vegetable, 1 fruit
> **Calories:** 150

STUFFED PEPPERS

1	green pepper	1
2 tablespoons	rice	30 milliliters
2 ounces	lean ground beef	60 grams
1	egg	1
1 teaspoon	onion flakes	5 milliliters
1 tablespoon	mushrooms (finely chopped)	15 milliliters
	salt & pepper to taste	
1 teaspoon	Tomato Sauce (page 168)	5 milliliters

Cut green pepper in half, lengthwise. Remove membrane and seeds; rinse, drain and reserve shells. Boil rice with ½ cup (125 milliliters) of water for 5 minutes; drain. Combine ground beef, rice, egg, onion flakes, and mushrooms; blend thoroughly. Add salt and pepper. Fill green pepper cavities with beef mixture; top with Tomato Sauce. Place in baking dish; cover. Bake at 350°F (175°C) for 20 to 25 minutes.

Microwave: Cook on HIGH for 10 minutes.

> **Yield:** 1 serving
> **Exchange:** 3 medium-fat meat, 1 bread, 1 vegetable
> **Calories:** 255

BEEF & RICE CASSEROLE

3 ounces	ground beef	90 grams
1 tablespoon	onion (chopped)	15 milliliters
1 tablespoon	celery (chopped)	15 milliliters
³/₄ cup	condensed chicken gumbo soup	180 milliliters
¹/₄ cup	water	60 milliliters
¹/₂ cup	rice (uncooked)	125 milliliters
¹/₄ cup	condensed cream of mushroom soup	60 milliliters
	salt & pepper to taste	

Combine ground beef, onion, and celery with a small amount of water in a saucepan. Boil until onion is tender; drain. Combine condensed chicken gumbo soup, water, and rice. Simmer until all moisture is absorbed. Mix beef mixture, rice, and mushroom soup; pour into a small greased casserole dish. Add salt and pepper. Bake at 350°F (175°C) for 25 minutes.

Microwave: Cook on MEDIUM for 8 to 10 minutes.

Yield:	1 serving
Exchange:	3 high-fat meat, 2 bread
Calories:	380

GERMAN GOULASH

3 ounces	lean ground beef	90 grams
1 teaspoon	onion chopped	5 milliliters
1 tablespoon	green pepper (chopped)	15 milliliters
1 tablespoon	celery (chopped)	15 milliliters
¹/₄	bay leaf (crushed)	¹/₄
¹/₂ cup	kidney beans (cooked)	125 milliliters
¹/₂ cup	elbow macaroni (cooked)	125 milliliters
¹/₄ cup	carrot (sliced)	60 milliliters
	salt & pepper to taste	

Brown ground beef, onion, green pepper, and celery over low heat; drain. Add crushed bay leaf, kidney beans, macaroni, and carrots; mix gently. Add salt and pepper. Pour into casserole dish; cover. Bake at 350°F (175°C) for 40 minutes.

Microwave: Cook on MEDIUM for 7 minutes.

Yield:	1 serving
Exchange:	3 medium-fat meat, 2¹/₂ bread
Calories:	413

CASSEROLES & ONE-DISH MEALS

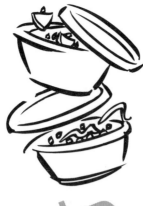

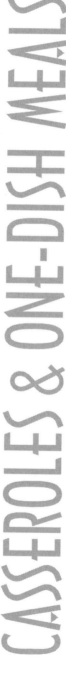

WIENER-EGG SCRAMBLE

1 slice	bacon	1 slice
1 teaspoon	onion (chopped)	5 milliliters
1	wiener (sliced)	1
1/2 teaspoon	green pepper (chopped)	2 milliliters
1	egg	1
1 teaspoon	skim milk	5 milliliters
dash	Worcestershire sauce	dash

Cook bacon until crisp; drain bacon and pan. Crumble bacon. Place bacon, onion, wiener, and green pepper in pan. Sauté on low heat until onion is tender. Beat egg with skim milk and Worcestershire sauce; pour over wiener mixture. Cook until set.

Yield: 1 serving
Exchange: 2 high-fat meat, 2 fat
Calories: 170

LASAGNE

2 ounces	ground beef	60 grams
1 tablespoon	onion (chopped)	15 milliliters
1/2 cup	Tomato Sauce (page 168)	125 milliliters
3 tablespoons	water	45 milliliters
1/4 teaspoon	garlic powder	1 milliliter
1/2 teaspoon	oregano	2 milliliters
	salt & pepper to taste	
1 1/2 cups	lasagne noodles (cooked)	375 milliliters
1 ounce	mozzarella cheese (grated)	30 grams
1 ounce	provolone cheese (grated)	30 grams

Crumble beef in small amount of water; add onion. Boil until meat is cooked; drain. Blend Tomato Sauce, 3 tablespoons (45 milliliters) water, garlic powder, oregano, salt, and pepper. Add beef-onion mixture; stir to blend. Spread small amount of sauce into bottom of individual baking dish. Layer noodles, sauce, mozzarella and provolone cheese. Bake at 375°F (190°C) for 30 minutes.

Microwave: Cook on HIGH for 10 minutes.

Yield: 1 serving
Exchange: 4 high-fat meat, 3 bread
Calories: 485

CHEESE LASAGNE

1/2 **cup**	Tomato Sauce (page 168)	125 milliliters
3 **tablespoons**	water	45 milliliters
1 **tablespoon**	onion	15 milliliters
1/4 **teaspoon**	garlic powder	1 milliliter
1/2 **teaspoon**	oregano	2 milliliters
	salt & pepper to taste	
1/4 **cup**	large curd cottage cheese	60 milliliters
1	egg	1
1 1/2 **cups**	lasagne noodles (cooked)	375 milliliters
2 **ounces**	mozzarella cheese	60 grams
1 **tablespoon**	Parmesan cheese	15 milliliters

Combine Tomato Sauce, water, onion, garlic powder, oregano, salt, and pepper. Thoroughly blend together cottage cheese and egg. Spread small amount of sauce into bottom of individual baking dish. Alternate layers of noodles, sauce, cottage cheese mixture, and mozzarella cheese. Top with Parmesan cheese. Bake at 375°F (190°C) for 30 minutes.

Microwave: Cook on HIGH for 10 minutes.

Yield: 1 serving
Exchange: 3 high-fat meat, 3 bread
Calories: 350

KOLE 'N KLUMP

1/2 **cup**	brussels sprouts	125 milliliters
2 **ounces**	lean pork cubes	60 grams
pinch	caraway seeds, salt, pepper	pinch
1/4 **cup**	potato (grated)	60 milliliters
1/4 **teaspoon**	onion salt	1 milliliter
dash each	thyme, salt, pepper,	dash each

Boil brussels sprouts, pork, caraway seeds, salt, and pepper with a small amount of water until partially cooked; drain. Place in individual baking dish. Cover with potato; sprinkle with onion salt, thyme, salt, and pepper. Cover tightly. Bake at 375°F (190°C) for 1 hour.

Microwave: Cook on HIGH for 10 to 12 minutes. Turn dish a quarter turn after 6 minutes.

Yield: 1 serving
Exchange: 1 bread, 2 high-fat meat
Calories: 232

CASSEROLES & ONE-DISH MEALS

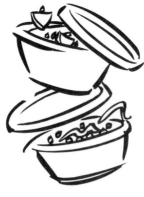

HAMBURGER PIE

2 pounds	lean ground beef	1 kilogram
¹/₂ cup	cornflakes (crushed)	125 milliliters
¹/₄ teaspoon	garlic powder	1 milliliter
¹/₂ teaspoon	onion (finely chopped)	2 milliliters
1	egg	1
	salt & pepper to taste	
2¹/₄ cups	water	560 milliliters
1 cup	skim milk	250 milliliters
1 teaspoon	salt	5 milliliters
2 cups	instant mashed potatoes	500 milliliters
1 teaspoon	margarine	5 milliliters

Combine ground beef, cornflakes, garlic powder, onion, and egg; mix well. Add salt and pepper. Place beef mixture in 9-inch (23-centimeter) pie pan. Pat to cover bottom and sides evenly. Bake at 425°F (220°C) for 30 minutes; drain off excess fat. Heat water, skim milk, and salt just to a boil; remove from heat. Add potato granules; mix thoroughly. Add margarine; blend well. Cover and allow to stand 5 minutes, or until potatoes thicken. Spread evenly over meat mixture. Return to oven and bake until potatoes are golden brown. Allow to rest 10 minutes before cutting pie into wedges.

Microwave: Cover beef mixture. Cook on MEDIUM for 10 to 12 minutes; drain. Cover with potatoes. Cook on MEDIUM for 2 minutes. Hold 5 minutes.

Yield:	8 servings
Exchange:	(1 serving) 4 high-fat meat, 1 bread, ¹/₂ fat
Calories:	(1 serving) 372

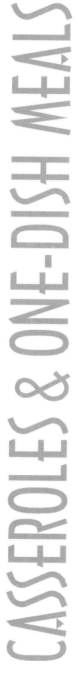

MACARONI AND CHEESE SUPREME

1 cup	elbow macaroni	250 milliliters
11-ounce can	condensed cream of mushroom soup	300-gram can
6 ounces	cheese (shredded)	180 milliliters
1 teaspoon	yellow mustard	5 milliliters
1 teaspoon	salt	5 milliliters
dash	pepper	dash
2 cups	cooked spinach (drained)	500 milliliters
12 ounces	lean meat (diced)	360 grams

Cook macaroni as directed on package; drain. Combine mushroom soup, cheese, mustard, salt, and pepper. Add macaroni; stir well. Spread cooked spinach on bottom of lightly greased 13 x 9-inch (33 x 23-centimeter) baking dish. Top with meat. Spoon macaroni mixture evenly over entire surface. Bake at 375°F (190°C) for 40 minutes. Allow to cool 15 minutes before serving.

Microwave: Cook on MEDIUM for 12 to 15 minutes. Turn dish halfway through cooking time. Allow to rest 15 minutes before serving.

Yield: 6 servings
Exchange: (1 serving) 2 bread, 3 high-fat meat, 1 vegetable
Calories: (1 serving) 287

HOT TUNA DISH

1/2 cup	condensed cream of chicken soup	125 milliliters
2 ounces	chunk tuna (in water)	60 grams
2 tablespoons	celery (diced)	30 milliliters
1 tablespoon	onion (chopped)	15 milliliters
1	egg (hard cooked)	1
4 tablespoons	potato chips (crushed)	60 milliliters

Combine condensed soup, tuna, celery, and onion; mix thoroughly. Pour into small casserole. Slice egg; layer egg, then crushed potato chips. Bake at 350°F (175°C) for 20 minutes.

Microwave: Cook on MEDIUM for 7 to 10 minutes.

Yield: 1 serving
Exchange: 1 1/3 bread, 3 medium-fat meat
Calories: 297

CASSEROLES & ONE-DISH MEALS

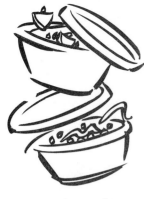

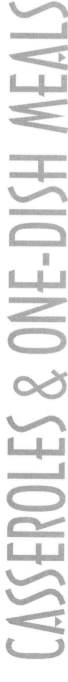

TURKEY À LA KING

1 tablespoon	green pepper (diced)	15 milliliters
2 tablespoons	celery (sliced)	30 milliliters
1/4 cup	condensed cream of chicken soup	60 milliliters
2 tablespoons	skim milk	30 milliliters
2 tablespoons	mushrooms (chopped)	30 milliliters
3 ounces	cooked turkey (diced)	90 grams
1 tablespoon	pimiento (chopped)	15 milliliters
	salt & pepper to taste	
2 slices	bread (toasted)	2 slices

Cook green pepper and celery in boiling water until tender; drain. Blend condensed soup and skim milk. Add green pepper, celery, mushrooms, turkey, and pimiento. Add salt and pepper. Heat slightly over low heat. Cut toast into triangles; place in small bowl, tips up. Spoon turkey mixture over tips.

Yield: 1 serving
Exchange: 3 medium-fat meat, 2 1/4 bread, 1/4 vegetable
Calories: 450

TURKEY À LA KING II

1/4 cup	White Sauce (page 164)	60 milliliters
1 ounce	cold turkey (diced)	30 grams
1/4 cup	mushroom pieces	60 milliliters
2 tablespoons	green pepper (chopped)	30 milliliters
1 tablespoon	stuffed green olives (chopped)	15 milliliters
	salt & pepper to taste	
	dough for 1 baking powder biscuit (page 141)	

Heat White Sauce. Combine sauce, turkey, mushrooms, green pepper, and olives; add salt and pepper. Pour into lightly greased individual baking dish. Top with biscuit dough. Bake at 375°F (190°C) for 15 to 20 minutes, or until biscuit is golden brown.

Yield: 1 serving
Exchange: 1 medium-fat meat, 1 vegetable, 1 bread
Calories: 168

MOSTACCIOLI WITH OYSTERS

8-ounce can	oysters with liquid (minced)	227-gram can
4-ounce can	mushroom pieces	120-gram can
1/2 cup	green pepper (sliced)	125 milliliters
1 tablespoon	parsley	15 milliliters
1 teaspoon	garlic powder	5 milliliters
	salt & pepper to taste	
3 cups	mostaccioli noodles (cooked)	750 milliliters

Combine minced oysters with liquid, mushrooms, green pepper, and parsley in saucepan. Add garlic powder. Cook until green pepper is crispy tender. Add salt and pepper. Serve over mostaccioli noodles.

Microwave: Combine minced oysters with liquid, mushrooms, green pepper, parsley, and garlic powder in bowl. Cook on HIGH for 4 minutes or until green pepper is crispy tender. Add salt and pepper. Serve over mostaccioli noodles.

> **Yield:** 2 servings
> **Exchange:** (1 serving) 4 lean meat, 1 1/2 bread
> **Calories:** (1 serving) 195

HAM & SCALLOPED POTATOES

2 ounces	lean ham (diced)	60 grams
1 medium	potato (peeled & sliced)	1 medium
2 tablespoons	onion	30 milliliters
2 teaspoons	parsley	10 milliliters
	vegetable cooking spray	
1/4 cup	condensed cream of celery soup	60 milliliters
1/4 cup	milk	60 milliliters
	salt & pepper to taste	

Combine ham, potato, onion, and parsley in baking dish coated with vegetable cooking spray. Blend condensed soup and milk; pour over potato mixture; cover. Bake at 350°F (175°C) for 1 hour, or until potatoes are tender. Add salt and pepper.

Microwave: Cook on HIGH for 10 minutes, or until potatoes are tender. Add salt and pepper.

> **Yield:** 1 serving
> **Exchange:** 2 high-fat meat, 1 1/2 bread, 1/2 milk
> **Calories:** 365

CASSEROLES & ONE-DISH MEALS

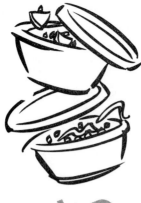

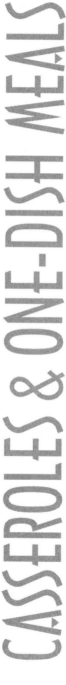

CHICKEN GAMBEANO

$^{1}/_{4}$ **cup**	condensed cream of chicken soup	60 milliliters
3 tablespoons	skim milk	45 milliliters
$^{1}/_{4}$ **cup**	zucchini (cubed)	60 milliliters
$^{1}/_{4}$ **cup**	green beans	60 milliliters
2 ounces	cooked chicken (cubed)	60 grams
$^{1}/_{4}$ **teaspoon**	poultry seasoning	1 milliliter
	salt & pepper to taste	
1$^{1}/_{4}$ cups	linguine (cooked)	310 milliliters

Blend condensed soup and skim milk; place in saucepan. Add zucchini and green beans. Cook over MEDIUM heat until vegetables are partially tender. Add chicken and seasonings; reheat. Serve over linguine.

Microwave: Blend condensed soup and skim milk in bowl. Add zucchini and green beans; cover. Cook on HIGH for 5 to 7 minutes, or until vegetables are partially tender. Add chicken and seasonings; reheat on MEDIUM for 4 minutes. Serve over linguine.

Yield:	1 serving
Exchange:	3 bread, 2 medium-fat meat, $^{1}/_{2}$ vegetable
Calories:	300

FISH NOODLE SPECIAL

$^{1}/_{4}$ **cup**	condensed cream of celery soup	60 milliliters
2 tablespoons	water	30 milliliters
2 tablespoons	mushroom pieces	30 milliliters
2 tablespoons	onion (finely chopped)	30 milliliters
dash each	thyme, ground rosemary, salt, pepper	dash each
1 cup	noodles (cooked)	250 milliliters
2 tablespoons	peas	30 milliliters
3 ounces	cooked perch (flaked)	90 grams

Blend condensed soup with water. Add mushrooms, onion, and seasonings; mix thoroughly. Combine noodles, peas, and perch in small baking dish. Pour soup mixture over entire surface; toss to mix. Bake at 350°F (175°C) for 30 minutes.

Microwave: Cook on HIGH for 5 to 6 minutes.

Yield:	1 serving
Exchange:	3 lean meat, 2$^{1}/_{2}$ bread
Calories:	285

TUNA SOUFFLÉ

11-ounce can	condensed cream of celery soup	300-gram can
2 teaspoons	parsley (finely chopped)	10 milliliters
1 teaspoon	salt	5 milliliters
dash	pepper	dash
1/2 teaspoon	marjoram	2 milliliters
7-ounce can	tuna (in water)	200-gram can
6	eggs (separated)	6
1 cup	mixed vegetables (cooked)	250 milliliters

Combine condensed soup, parsley, salt, pepper, marjoram, and tuna in saucepan. Heat, stirring constantly, until mixture is hot. Remove from heat and cool slightly. Add egg yolks, one at a time, beating well after each addition. Stir in vegetables. Beat egg whites until soft peaks form. Fold small amount of beaten egg whites into egg yolk mixture, then fold egg yolk mixture into remaining egg whites. Pour into lightly greased 10-inch (25-centimeter) soufflé dish. Bake at 325°F (165°C) for 50 minutes, or until firm and golden brown. Serve immediately.

Yield: 8 servings
Exchange: (1 serving) 1 1/2 lean meat, 1 bread
Calories: (1 serving) 134

CASSEROLE OF SHRIMP

2 teaspoons	margarine	10 milliliters
1 tablespoon	parsley (chopped)	15 milliliters
1 tablespoon	sherry	15 milliliters
dash each	garlic powder, paprika, cayenne	dash each
1/2 cup	soft bread crumbs	125 milliliters
3 ounces	large shrimp (cooked)	90 grams

Melt margarine over low heat. Add parsley, sherry, and seasonings; cook slightly. Add bread crumbs; toss to mix. Place shrimp in small baking dish. Top with bread crumb mixture. Bake at 325°F (165°C) for 20 minutes.

Microwave: Melt margarine; add parsley, sherry, and seasonings. Cook on HIGH for 2 minutes. Add bread crumbs; toss to mix. Place shrimp in small baking dish. Top with bread crumb mixture. Cook on MEDIUM for 5 to 7 minutes.

Yield: 1 serving
Exchange: 3 high-fat meat, 1 bread
Calories: 204

CASSEROLES & ONE-DISH MEALS

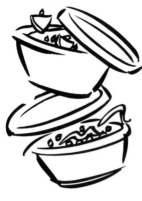

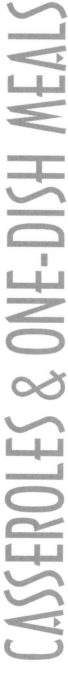

VEAL STEAK PARMESAN

1 tablespoon	flour	15 milliliters
1 teaspoon	salt	5 milliliters
dash each	poultry seasoning, salt, pepper, paprika	dash each
4 ounces	veal steak (cut in half)	120 grams
1 teaspoon	shortening	5 milliliters
1/2 cup	wide noodles (cooked)	125 milliliters
1/2 cup	Sour Cream Sauce (prepared)	125 milliliters
3 tablespoons	hot water	45 milliliters
1 teaspoon	Parmesan cheese	5 milliliters

Combine flour, salt, and seasonings in shaker bag. Add veal steak; shake to coat. Remove veal from bag and shake off excess flour. Heat shortening in small skillet. Brown veal on both sides; place in small baking dish. Cover with noodles. Blend Sour Cream Sauce and hot water. Pour over noodles. Top with Parmesan cheese. Bake at 350°F (175°C) for 45 minutes, or until veal is tender.

Microwave: Cover. Cook on MEDIUM to HIGH for 15 minutes, or until meat is tender.

Yield: 1 serving
Exchange: 4 1/4 medium-fat meat, 2 bread
Calories: 390

HUNGARIAN GOULASH

1 tablespoon	shortening or margarine	15 milliliters
1 ounce	lean beef (diced)	30 grams
1 ounce	lean veal (diced)	30 grams
1 ounce	beef kidney (diced)	30 grams
2 teaspoons	onion (chopped)	10 milliliters
1 teaspoon	green pepper (chopped)	5 milliliters
3	cherry tomatoes (halved)	3
1/2 cup	potato (diced)	125 milliliters
1/4 cup	carrot (diced)	60 milliliters
1/4 teaspoon	salt	1 milliliter
dash each	paprika, pepper, marjoram	dash each

Heat shortening or margarine in skillet; add meat. Brown on all sides; drain. Place in individual casserole. Add remaining ingredients. Add enough water to cover. Cover casserole tightly; bake at 350°F (175°C) for 1 hour.

Microwave: Cook on HIGH for 20 to 25 minutes. Stir halfway through cooking time.

Yield:	1 serving	
Exchange:	3 high-fat meat, 1 bread, 1 vegetable	
Calories:	348	

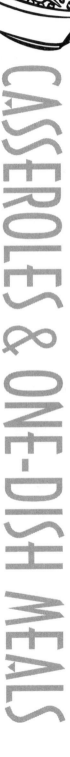

STUFFED CABBAGE ROLLS

2 large	cabbage leaves	2 large
2 ounces	ground veal	60 grams
2 ounces	ground lean beef	60 grams
3 tablespoons	skim milk	45 milliliters
1 slice	dry bread (crumbled)	1 slice
1 teaspoon	onion (grated)	5 milliliters
dash each	salt, pepper, nutmeg	dash each
1/2 cup	beef broth	125 milliliters
1 tablespoon	flour	15 milliliters

Cook cabbage leaves in boiling salted water until tender; drain. Combine ground veal, beef, skim milk, bread crumbs, onion, salt, pepper, and nutmeg; mix thoroughly. Place half of meat mixture in a cabbage leaf and roll up, tucking ends in. Secure with toothpicks. Place in small baking dish. Repeat with remaining meat mixture and cabbage leaf. Blend beef broth and flour; pour over cabbage rolls. Bake at 350°F (175°C) for 45 to 50 minutes.

Microwave: Cook on MEDIUM for 10 to 12 minutes.

Yield:	1 serving	
Exchange:	4 medium-fat meat, 1 vegetable, 1 bread	
Calories:	396	

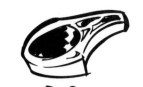

STEAK ROBERTO

¹/₄ **cup**	margarine	60 milliliters
1 teaspoon	garlic powder	5 milliliters
1 pound	beef tenderloin (8 slices)	500 grams
¹/₂ **teaspoon**	steak sauce	2 milliliters
¹/₄ **teaspoon**	bay leaf (crushed)	1 millilitre
1 tablespoon	lemon juice	15 milliliters
¹/₂ **teaspoon**	salt	2 milliliters
dash	pepper	dash

Melt margarine and combine with garlic powder. Set aside for 20 minutes to allow flavor to develop. Heat 1 tablespoon (15 milliliters) of the garlic margarine in heavy skillet until very hot. Place as many beef tenderloin slices as possible in skillet; brown on both sides. Remove to warm steak platter. Repeat with remaining beef, if necessary. Reduce heat. Add remaining garlic margarine to pan. Add steak sauce, bay leaf, lemon juice, salt, and pepper; blend thoroughly. Pour over beef tenderloin on platter.

Yield: 8 servings
Exchange: (1 serving) 2 medium-fat meat, ¹/₂ fat
Calories: (1 serving) 155

BRISKET OF BEEF WITH HORSERADISH

3 to 4 pounds	beef brisket	1¹/₂ to 2 kilograms
	salt & pepper to taste	
1 medium	onion (sliced)	1 medium
1	bay leaf	1
1 tablespoon	lemon juice	15 milliliters
¹/₂ **cup**	horseradish (grated)	125 milliliters
	salt & pepper to taste	

Place brisket in large kettle; add salt and pepper. Add onion, bay leaf, and enough water to cover brisket. Bring to a boil. Reduce heat and simmer for 2 hours. Remove brisket from water. Combine lemon juice and horseradish. Rub surface of brisket with horseradish mixture. Return brisket to kettle; cover. Cook 1 hour longer.

Exchange: (1 ounce/30 grams) 1 medium-fat meat
Calories: (1 ounce/30 grams) 84

BEEF FONDUE

1 small	tomato	1 small
2 cups	beef broth	500 milliliters
1	bay leaf	1
1/2 teaspoon	rosemary (ground)	2 milliliters
	sirloin steak (cut into bite-size cubes)	

Peel and crush tomato. Place beef broth, tomato, bay leaf, and rosemary in saucepan; heat to a boil. Pour into fondue pot, keep hot with a burner. Place steak cubes on spear. Cook in hot broth to desired doneness.

Exchange: (1 ounce/30 grams) 1 high-fat meat
Calories: (1 ounce/30 grams) 88

Note: Amount of steak used depends on number of servings required.

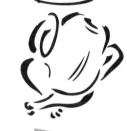

MEATS & POULTRY

SAUERBRATEN

4 ounces	lean beef roast	120 grams
1/2 cup	beef broth	125 milliliters
1/4 cup	water	60 milliliters
1/4 cup	cider vinegar	60 milliliters
1/4 teaspoon	salt	1 milliliter
dash	garlic powder	dash
1 teaspoon	margarine	5 milliliters

Place beef in glass pan or bowl. Combine remaining ingredients, except margarine; pour over beef. Marinate 4 to 5 days in refrigerator. Turn beef at least once a day. Melt margarine in small skillet; add beef and brown. Reduce heat. Add half of the marinade to the skillet. Simmer until beef is tender.

Yield: 1 serving
Exchange: 4 medium-fat meat
Calories: 300

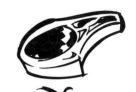

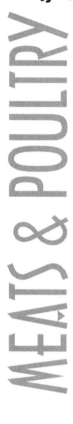

MUSHROOM-STUFFED PORK CHOPS

2 tablespoons	mushroom pieces	30 milliliters
1 teaspoon	onion (chopped)	5 milliliters
1/2 teaspoon	parsley (chopped)	2 milliliters
1 teaspoon	raisins (soaked)	5 milliliters
1/4 teaspoon	nutmeg	1 milliliter
1	double pork chop	1

Combine ingredients for stuffing; stir to blend. Split meaty part of chop down to bone; do not split through bone. Fill with stuffing; secure with poultry pins. Place on baking sheet. Bake uncovered at 350°F (175°C) for 35 to 40 minutes, or until tender. Turn once.

Yield: 1 chop
Exchange: (1 ounce/30 grams) 1 high-fat meat
Calories: (1 ounce/30 grams) 109

TERIYAKI PORK STEAK

	pork steak (thinly sliced)	
1/2 cup	soy sauce	125 milliliters
1 tablespoon	wine vinegar	15 milliliters
2 tablespoons	lemon juice	30 milliliters
1/4 cup	water	60 milliliters
2 tablespoons	sugar replacement	30 milliliters
1 1/2 teaspoons	ginger	7 milliliters
1/2 teaspoon	garlic powder	2 milliliters

Place slices of pork steak in shallow dish. Combine remaining ingredients; pour over pork. Marinate 1 to 2 hours; turn once. Broil pork 5 to 6 inches (12 to 15 centimeters) from heat, for 2 to 3 minutes per side. Turn and broil second side.

Exchange: (1 ounce/30 grams) 1 medium-fat meat
Calories: (1 ounce/30 grams) 89

Note: Amount of steak used depends on number of servings required.

CALF'S LIVER

1 tablespoon	flour	15 milliliters
¹/₂ teaspoon	bay leaf (finely crushed)	2 milliliters
¹/₄ teaspoon	nutmeg	1 milliliter
	salt & pepper to taste	
¹/₂ cup	beef broth	125 milliliters
3 ounces	calf's liver (remove any membrane)	90 grams
	vegetable cooking spray	

Combine flour, bay leaf, nutmeg, salt, and pepper in shaker bag. Add liver; shake to coat. Remove liver from bag and shake off excess flour. Brown liver in heavy skillet coated with vegetable cooking spray. Reduce heat. Add beef broth; cover. Simmer for 25 to 30 minutes, or until tender.

Yield: 1 serving
Exchange: 3 lean meat
Calories: 132

CALF'S BRAINS

1	calf's brain (trimmed)	1
2 tablespoons	lemon juice	30 milliliters
1 tablespoon	cider vinegar	15 milliliters
1 teaspoon	thyme	5 milliliters
1	bay leaf	1
¹/₃ cup	onion (chopped)	90 milliliters
1	parsley sprig (chopped)	1
¹/₃ cup	celery (chopped)	90 milliliters

Rinse brain thoroughly. Cover with water. Add lemon juice and marinate for 2 to 4 hours. Drain. Cover with cold water. Add remaining ingredients. Bring to boil. Cover and simmer for 20 to 25 minutes, or until thoroughly cooked. Remove from heat. Allow to rest 15 minutes. Remove brain from water. Slice thin.

Yield: 1 brain
Exchange: (1 ounce/30 grams) 1 lean meat
Calories: (1 ounce/30 grams) 45

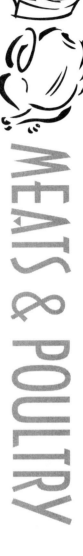

MEATS & POULTRY

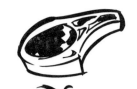

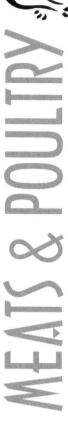
VEAL ROAST

2 to 3 pounds	veal roast	1 to 1½ kilograms
2 cups	beef broth	500 milliliters
1 medium	onion (sliced)	1 medium
1	bay leaf	1
¼ teaspoon	thyme	1 milliliter
	salt & pepper to taste	

Place roast in heavy kettle or roasting pan. Combine remaining ingredients. Pour over roast. Bake at 375°F (190°C) for 2 to 2½ hours, or until meat is very tender. While baking, baste with pan juices.

> **Exchange:** (1 ounce/30 grams) 1 lean meat
> **Calories:** (1 ounce/30 grams) 55

VEAL SCALOPPINE

2 ounces	veal steak (boned)	60 grams
¼ cup	tomato (sieved)	60 milliliters
2 tablespoons	green pepper (chopped)	30 milliliters
1 tablespoon	mushroom pieces	15 milliliters
1 tablespoon	onions (chopped)	15 milliliters
¼ teaspoon	parsley	1 milliliter
dash each	garlic powder, oregano	dash each
	salt & pepper to taste	

Place veal on bottom of individual baking dish. Add remaining ingredients; cover. Bake at 350°F (175°C) for 45 minutes, or until meat is tender.

Microwave: Cook on HIGH for 10 to 12 minutes. Turn and uncover last 2 minutes.

> **Yield:** 1 serving
> **Exchange:** 2 lean meat, 1 vegetable
> **Calories:** 164

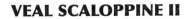

VEAL SCALOPPINE II

2 ounces	veal round steak (thinly sliced)	60 grams
1/2 teaspoon	margarine	2 milliliters
2 tablespoons	tomato paste	30 milliliters
6 tablespoons	water	90 milliliters
dash each	salt, pepper, oregano, garlic powder	dash each
1 tablespoon	mushrooms (sliced)	15 milliliters
1 teaspoon	onion (chopped)	5 milliliters
1 cup	spaghetti (cooked)	250 milliliters

Melt margarine in small skillet. Brown both sides of slices of veal steak. Place in small baking dish. Blend tomato paste, water, seasonings, mushrooms, and onion together. Pour over veal; cover. Bake at 350°F (175°C) for 30 minutes. Place veal on top of spaghetti. Pour sauce over all.

Microwave: Cook covered on MEDIUM for 12 minutes.

Yield: 1 serving
Exchange: 2 medium-fat meat, 2 bread
Calories: 310

VEAL ROLL

1 ounce	veal (thin slice)	30 grams
	salt & pepper to taste	
1/2 ounce	prosciutto (thin slice)	15 grams
1/2 ounce	Swiss cheese (thin slice)	15 grams
	vegetable cooking spray	

Pound veal slice with mallet or edge of plate until very thin. Add salt and pepper. Place prosciutto on top and roll up. Secure with poultry pin. Brown in heavy skillet coated with vegetable cooking spray. Top with cheese slice. Cover. Cook over low heat just until cheese melts slightly. Serve on hot plate.

Yield: 1 serving
Exchange: 2 medium-fat meat
Calories: 156

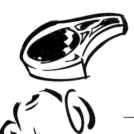

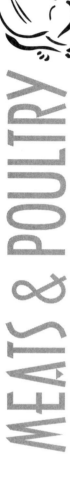

BEEF TONGUE

1	beef tongue	1

Place tongue in large kettle; cover with water. Add 1 teaspoon (5 milliliters) salt per quart (liter) of water. Bring to boil; reduce heat and simmer 3½ to 4 hours. Remove tongue; immediately place in ice water. Allow to soak 5 minutes. Remove skin and trim. Slice thin. Use for sandwiches.

Exchange: (1 ounce/30 grams) 1 lean meat
Calories: (1 ounce/30 grams) 51

KLIP KLOPS

4 slices	bread (crust removed)	4 slices
½ cup	skim milk	125 milliliters
½ teaspoon	garlic powder	2 milliliters
1 teaspoon	onion salt	5 milliliters
1 pound	lean ground beef	500 grams
1	egg (beaten)	1
1 quart	water	1 liter
1 small	bay leaf	1 small
1 teaspoon	salt	5 milliliters
1	clove	1

Soak bread in skim milk. Add garlic powder, onion salt, ground beef, and egg; mix thoroughly. Form into 8 balls. Combine water, bay leaf, salt, and clove. Bring to boil. Drop balls into boiling water. Cook until beef is done (about 15 minutes). Drain before placing on hot platter.

Yield: 8 servings
Exchange: (1 serving) 2 high-fat meat, 1 bread
Calories: (1 serving) 190

MEAT LOAF

2 pounds	lean ground beef	1 kilogram
¼ cup	onion (grated)	60 milliliters
1 cup	soft bread crumbs	250 milliliters
1	egg	1
¼ cup	parsley (finely snipped)	60 milliliters
1¼ teaspoons	salt	6 milliliters
dash each	pepper, thyme; marjoram	dash each
1 teaspoon	evaporated milk	5 milliliters

Combine all ingredients. Add just enough water to form firm ball. Press into baking dish. Bake at 350°F (175°C) for 1½ hours.

Microwave: Cook on HIGH for 15 minutes. Turn dish halfway through cooking time. Allow to rest for 5 minutes before serving.

> **Yield:** 12 servings
> **Exchange:** (1 serving) 2½ high-fat meat, ¼ bread
> **Calories:** (1 serving) 237

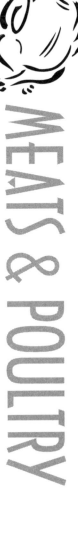

ROAST LEG OF LAMB

5- to 6-pound	leg of lamb	2½- to 3-kilogram
½ cup	lo-cal Italian dressing	125 milliliters
½ cup	water	125 milliliters
3 tablespoons	lemon juice	45 milliliters
1 teaspoon	garlic powder	5 milliliters
½ teaspoon	rosemary (ground)	2 milliliters
½ teaspoon	thyme	2 milliliters
½ teaspoon	mace	2 milliliters
1 teaspoon	salt	5 milliliters
¼ teaspoon	pepper	1 milliliter

Wipe lamb with damp cloth. Puncture lamb with long sharp spear or poultry pin. Place on a rack in roasting pan, fat side up. Blend remaining ingredients; pour over lamb. Roast uncovered at 325°F (165°C) for 3 to 3½ hours. Baste with pan juices every half hour. Add more Italian dressing and water, if necessary.

> **Exchange:** (1 ounce/30 grams) 1 medium-fat meat
> **Calories:** (1 ounce/30 grams) 75

MEATS & POULTRY

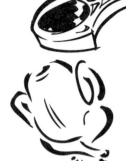

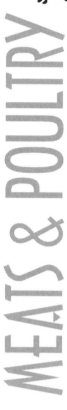

STEAK HAWAIIAN

3 ounces	beef top round steak (sliced)	90 grams
¹/₂ teaspoon	mace	2 milliliters
2 tablespoons	unsweetened pineapple juice	30 milliliters
1	pineapple slice (unsweetened)	1

Pound slices of round steak with mallet or edge of plate until thin. Sprinkle both sides with mace. Place in aluminum foil. Sprinkle with pineapple juice; top with pineapple slice. Secure foil tightly. Place in baking dish. Bake at 350°F (175°C) for 40 to 45 minutes.

Microwave: Place in plastic wrap. Cook on HIGH for 10 to 12 minutes.

Yield: 1 serving
Exchange: 3 lean meat, 1 fruit
Calories: 200

LAMB SHISH KEBAB

4 pounds	lean lamb	2 kilograms
3	garlic cloves (crushed)	3
1¹/₂ teaspoons	salt	7 milliliters
1	bay leaf	1
¹/₂ teaspoon	pepper	2 milliliters
¹/₂ teaspoon	ground allspice	2 milliliters
¹/₂ teaspoon	ground clove	2 milliliters
1 teaspoon	white vinegar	5 milliliters
1 cup	skim milk	250 milliliters

Cut lamb into 2-inch (5-centimeter) cubes. Combine remaining ingredients; blend thoroughly. Pour over lamb in large bowl; cover. Refrigerate overnight. Place lamb pieces on skewers. Barbecue or broil 10 to 15 minutes. Turn once.

Exchange: (1 ounce/30 grams) 1 medium-fat meat
Calories: (1 ounce/30 grams) 89

SWISS STEAK

3 ounces	beef minute steak	90 grams
	salt & pepper to taste	
1 teaspoon	margarine	5 milliliters
¼ cup	celery (sliced)	60 milliliters
1 tablespoon	onion (chopped)	15 milliliters
¼ cup	tomato (crushed)	60 milliliters
¼ cup	water	60 milliliters

Heat margarine until very hot. Salt and pepper the steak. Brown both sides; drain. Place in individual baking dish. Add salt, pepper, and remaining ingredients. Cover. Bake at 375°F (190°C) for 1 hour, or until steak is tender.

Microwave: Cook on HIGH for 8 to 10 minutes. Uncover last minute.

Yield:	1 serving
Exchange:	3 medium-fat meat, 1 fat
Calories:	220

ROAST DUCK WITH ORANGE SAUCE

4- to 5-pound	duck	2- to 3-kilogram
2 medium	oranges	2 medium
	salt to taste	
	Orange Sauce (page 165)	

Wash inside and outside of duck thoroughly. Remove any fat from tail or neck opening. Salt interior of bird. Cut each orange (with peel) into 8 sections. Place inside of duck. Secure tail and neck skin, legs and wings with poultry pins. Salt exterior of duck. Place breast side up on a rack in roasting pan. Bake at 350°F (175°C) for 4 hours. During the final hour, baste with Orange Sauce every 15 minutes.

Exchange:	(1 ounce/30 grams) 1 high-fat meat
Calories:	(1 ounce/30 grams) 96

MEATS & POULTRY

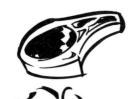

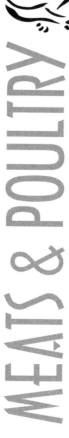

ROAST GOOSE

5- to 6-pound	goose	2½- to 3-kilogram
	salt to taste	

Wash and dry goose thoroughly. Salt cavity and exterior. Fill cavity loosely with stuffing. Close cavity and secure tightly. Place breast side up in roasting pan. Roast at 350°F (175°C) for 30 to 40 minutes per pound, or about 3 to 4 hours. Cover with a loose tent of aluminum foil for the last hour to prevent excess browning.

Yield:	8 to 10 servings
Exchange:	(1 ounce/30 grams) 1 high-fat meat (without skin)
Calories:	(1 ounce/30 grams) 120 (without skin)

Note: Add exchanges and calories for stuffing.

POLLO LESSO

3 ounces	chicken breast (boned)	90 grams
½	tomato (cut in 4 pieces)	½
¼	cucumber (peeled and sliced)	¼
¼ cup	peas	60 milliliters
dash each	salt, pepper, parsley	dash each

Remove skin from chicken breast; boil chicken in small amount of salted water until almost tender. Add tomato pieces, cucumber slices, and peas. Heat thoroughly; drain. Place on serving plate. Sprinkle with salt, pepper, and parsley.

Microwave: Place skinned chicken breast in individual dish; cover with plastic wrap. Cook on HIGH for 12 minutes. Drain off any moisture. Add vegetables. Sprinkle with salt, pepper, and parsley. Cook on MEDIUM for 4 minutes.

Yield:	1 serving
Exchange:	3 lean meat, 1 bread
Calories:	202

EL DORADO

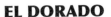

1 ounce	cooked chicken (diced)	30 grams
¹/₂ cup	chicken broth	125 milliliters
¹/₂ ounce	fresh oysters	15 grams
1 teaspoon	margarine	5 milliliters
1 tablespoon	carrot (grated)	15 milliliters
2 tablespoons	celery (chopped)	30 milliliters
1 teaspoon	parsley (chopped)	5 milliliters
	salt & pepper to taste	

Heat chicken broth to a boil; add oysters. Cook until edges roll; drain. Heat margarine in heavy skillet. Add carrot, celery, and parsley. Sauté until crisp-tender. Add chicken, oysters, and 1 tablespoon (15 milliliters) of the chicken broth. Cook until thoroughly heated. Drain, if necessary. Add salt and pepper.

Yield: 1 serving
Exchange: 1¹/₂ lean meat, 2 fat
Calories: 80

CHICKEN LIVERS

3 ounces	chicken livers	90 grams
¹/₂ cup	skim milk	125 milliliters
2 tablespoons	flour	30 milliliters
2 teaspoons	margarine	10 milliliters
	salt & pepper to taste	

Soak chicken livers in skim milk overnight. Drain. Combine flour, salt, and pepper in shaker bag. Add livers, one at a time; shake to coat. Remove livers from bag and shake off excess flour. Melt margarine in small skillet; add livers. Cook until lightly browned and tender.

Yield: 1 serving
Exchange: 3 lean meat, 2 fat
Calories: 190

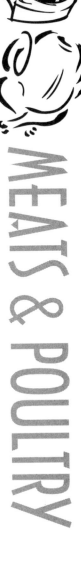

MEATS & POULTRY

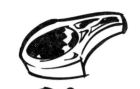

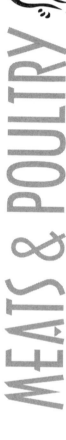

MEATS & POULTRY

GIBLET-STUFFED CHICKEN

3 ounces	chicken breast (skinned & boned)	90 grams
2	giblets	2
1 teaspoon	margarine	5 milliliters
2 tablespoons	rice	30 milliliters
1 tablespoon	raisins	15 milliliters
1 tablespoon	unsalted peanuts	15 milliliters
	salt & pepper to taste	

Simmer giblets in boiling water for 1 hour, or until tender. Remove tough center core from giblets. Chop giblets into small pieces. Melt margarine in small skillet. Sauté rice, raisins, giblets, and peanuts until rice and giblets are golden brown. Remove from heat. Add salt and pepper. Add ¼ cup (60 milliliters) water. Cover and return to heat. Simmer for 15 minutes or until water is absorbed. Remove from heat. Remove cover and allow to cool slightly. Place chicken breast, boned side up, between two sheets of plastic wrap or waxed paper. Pound from center with the heel of your hand or edge of a plate to flatten. Place dressing in center. Fold over and secure with toothpicks or poultry pins. Place in small baking dish. Bake in preheated over at 350°F (175°C) for 1 hour, or until golden brown.

Microwave: Sprinkle with paprika and parsley. Cook on HIGH for 18 minutes.

> **Yield:** 1 serving
> **Exchange:** 3½ lean meat, ½ fruit, ¼ bread, 1½ fat
> **Calories:** 255

SWEET PORK & RAISIN BRAN
BREAKFAST SAUSAGE

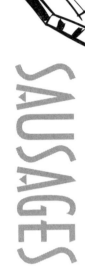

1/2 cup	ice-cold orange juice	125 milliliters
1/2 teaspoon	celery flakes	2 milliliters
1/4 teaspoon	ground nutmeg	1 milliliter
3/4 teaspoon	ground black pepper	4 milliliters
1/2 teaspoon	ground sage	2 milliliters
3/4 teaspoon	salt	4 milliliters
1/4 teaspoon	ground thyme	1 milliliter
1 pound	freshly ground pork	500 grams
1 1/2 cups	raisin bran flakes	375 milliliters

Pour orange juice into a large bowl. Add seasonings and stir. Add ground pork and raisin bran flakes. Follow directions below.

Yield: 16 servings
Exchange: (1 serving) 1 medium-fat meat
Calories: (1 serving) 80

DIRECTIONS FOR ALL SAUSAGES

Mix sausage the old-fashioned way with *clean hands* until *thoroughly* blended. Wrap sausage in plastic and refrigerate for several hours or overnight to allow herbs, spices and seasonings to permeate the meat. Sausage can be formed into patties or stuffed into natural casings, using standard stuffing procedures. Make 16 patties or links per recipe unless recipe specifies 8 patties or links. Fresh pork sausage should be refrigerated and used within a day or 2. Pan-fry or bake sausage until brown and juicy. *Pork must be cooked thoroughly.* Cooked or uncooked sausage can be individually wrapped with waxed paper, placed in a freezer bag and frozen for future use.

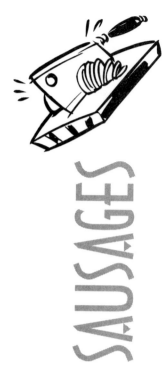

SWEET BEEF WITH APPLES
BREAKFAST SAUSAGE

1/2 cup	ice-cold apple juice	125 milliliters
1/2 teaspoon	ground cinnamon	2 milliliters
1/2 teaspoon	parsley flakes	2 milliliters
1/4 teaspoon	ground marjoram	1 milliliter
3/4 teaspoon	ground black pepper	4 milliliters
1/2 teaspoon	ground sage	2 milliliters
3/4 teaspoon	salt	4 milliliters
1 pound	freshly ground beef	500 grams
1 cup	uncooked oatmeal	250 milliliters
3 tablespoons	dried apple (diced)	45 milliliters

Pour apple juice into large bowl. Add seasonings and stir. Add ground beef, oatmeal and dried apple. Mix sausage the old-fashioned way, following directions on page 109.

Yield: 16 servings
Exchange: (1 serving) 1 lean meat
Calories: (1 serving) 46

HOT PORK BREAKFAST SAUSAGE

1	egg	1
1/4 cup	ice-cold tomato juice	60 milliliters
1/4 teaspoon	ground allspice	1 milliliter
1/4 teaspoon	ground basil	1 milliliter
1/2 teaspoon	parsley flakes	2 milliliters
1/4 teaspoon	ground ginger	1 milliliter
1 teaspoon	ground paprika	5 milliliters
3/4 teaspoon	cayenne pepper	4 milliliters
1/4 teaspoon	cayenne pepper flakes	1 milliliter
1/2 teaspoon	ground sage	2 milliliters
1/2 teaspoon	salt	2 milliliters
1 pound	freshly ground pork	500 grams
1 cup	wheat germ	250 milliliters

In a large bowl, combine egg and tomato juice. Blend seasonings into the liquid. Add pork and wheat germ. Mix sausage the old-fashioned way, following directions on page 109.

Yield: 16 servings
Exchange: (1 serving) 1 high-fat meat
Calories: (1 serving) 93

Added touch: Although this is an excellent breakfast sausage, it's *great* at a picnic when grilled on an outdoor charcoal barbecue and served on a bun.

Yield: 8 servings
Exchange: (1 serving) 2 high-fat meat
Calories: (1 serving) 187

Note: Add exchanges and calories for bun and condiments.

HOT BEEF BREAKFAST SAUSAGE

1	egg	1
¹/₄ cup	ice-cold mixed vegetable juice	60 milliliters
¹/₂ teaspoon	celery seed	2 milliliters
¹/₄ teaspoon	ground mustard	1 milliliter
¹/₄ teaspoon	ground oregano	1 milliliter
1 teaspoon	ground paprika	5 milliliters
¹/₂ teaspoon	cayenne pepper	2 milliliters
¹/₂ teaspoon	cayenne pepper flakes	2 milliliters
¹/₂ teaspoon	ground sage	2 milliliters
¹/₂ teaspoon	salt	2 milliliters
1 pound	freshly ground beef	500 grams
1¹/₂ cups	40% bran flakes	375 milliliters

Combine egg and vegetable juice in a large bowl and blend in the seasonings. Add ground beef and bran flakes. Mix sausage the old-fashioned way, following directions on page 109.

Yield: 16 servings
Exchange: (1 serving) 1 lean-fat meat
Calories: (1 serving) 51

Added touch: Although this is an excellent breakfast sausage, it is scrumptious at a picnic when grilled on an outdoor charcoal barbecue and served on a bun.

Yield: 8 servings
Exchange: (1 serving) 1 high-fat meat
Calories: (1 serving) 102

Note: Add exchanges and calories for bun and condiments.

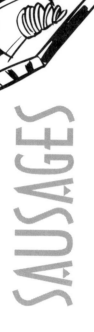

SWEET MINTED LAMB
BREAKFAST SAUSAGE

¹/₂ **cup**	ice-cold pineapple juice	125 milliliters
¹/₄ **teaspoon**	ground cinnamon	1 milliliter
¹/₂ **teaspoon**	dried mint flakes	2 milliliters
¹/₄ **teaspoon**	ground marjoram	1 milliliter
³/₄ **teaspoon**	ground black pepper	4 milliliters
¹/₄ **teaspoon**	ground rosemary	1 milliliter
¹/₂ **teaspoon**	ground sage	2 milliliters
³/₄ **teaspoon**	salt	4 milliliters
¹/₄ **teaspoon**	ground thyme	1 milliliter
1 pound	freshly ground lamb	500 grams
1 cup	yellow cornmeal	250 milliliters

In a large bowl, blend pineapple juice and seasonings. Add ground lamb and cornmeal. Mix sausage the old-fashioned way, following directions on page 109.

Yield: 16 servings
Exchange: (1 serving) 1 lean meat
Calories: (1 serving) 53

GERMAN-STYLE BRATWURST

Bratwurst is a plump traditional sausage that originated in Nürnberg, Germany. In the German language, *brat* means "to fry" and *wurst* means "sausage." Bratwurst, well-known throughout the world, is a common cookout favorite in the United States Midwest, especially in the Sheboygan/Milwaukee, Wisconsin area.

Bratwurst can be made of pork, beef and/or veal. There are countless ways to make bratwurst. Each sausagemaker *(wurstmacher)* blends his or her own bratwurst variation, according to personal, regional and ethnic preferences. Bratwurst tastes best when charcoal-grilled and served with your favorite condiments on a German-style bun. The following bratwurst recipes are only a sampling of the hundreds of delightful variations that bratwurst fans have created. Although bratwurst is usually an all-meat sausage, these high-fiber variations retain the authentic style and flavor of the original recipes.

SMOKEY-STYLE PORK BRATWURST

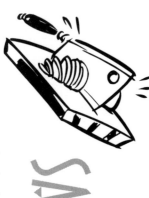

1	egg	1
¹/₄ cup	ice water	60 milliliters
1 teaspoon	liquid smoke	5 milliliters
1 teaspoon	caraway seeds	5 milliliters
¹/₂ teaspoon	celery flakes	2 milliliters
¹/₄ teaspoon	parsley flakes	1 milliliter
¹/₄ teaspoon	ground ginger	1 milliliter
¹/₂ teaspoon	ground dry orange peel	2 milliliters
¹/₄ teaspoon	ground nutmeg	1 milliliter
1 teaspoon	onion powder	5 milliliters
¹/₂ teaspoon	ground white pepper	2 milliliters
³/₄ teaspoon	salt	4 milliliters
¹/₄ teaspoon	brown sugar	1 milliliter
1 pound	freshly ground pork	500 grams
1¹/₄ cups	40% bran flakes	310 milliliters

In a large bowl, combine the egg, water and liquid smoke. Crush caraway seeds, celery and parsley flakes with a mortar and pestle. Blend all seasonings into the liquid. Add pork and bran flakes. Mix sausage the old-fashioned way, following directions on page 109. Make eight patties or links per recipe.

Added touch: Bake fresh or frozen bratwurst with sauerkraut for a delectable main dish.

Yield:	8 servings
Exchange:	(1 serving) 2 medium-fat meat
Calories:	(1 serving) 151

SMOKEY-STYLE BEEF AND PORK BRATWURST

1	egg	1
1 teaspoon	liquid smoke	5 milliliters
¼ cup	ice water	60 milliliters
¼ teaspoon	allspice	1 milliliter
½ teaspoon	caraway seeds	2 milliliters
1½ teaspoons	celery flakes	7 milliliters
¼ teaspoon	ground ginger	1 milliliter
1 teaspoon	ground dry lemon peel	5 milliliters
¼ teaspoon	ground mace	1 milliliter
1 teaspoon	onion flakes	5 milliliters
¾ teaspoon	ground black pepper	4 milliliters
¾ teaspoon	salt	4 milliliters
dash	brown sugar	dash
½ pound	freshly ground beef	250 grams
½ pound	freshly ground pork	250 grams
1 cup	wheat germ	250 milliliters

Add egg, liquid smoke and water to large bowl. Crush caraway seeds and celery flakes in a mortar with pestle. Blend seasonings into the liquid. Add beef, pork and wheat germ. Mix sausage the old-fashioned way, following directions on page 109. Make eight patties or links per recipe.

Added touch: Use diced, sliced or crumbled bratwurst as a pizza topping.

Yield: 8 servings
Exchange: (1 serving) 2 medium-fat meat
Calories: (1 serving) 169

Note: Add exchanges and calories of pizza dough and other toppings.

SPICY BEEF BRATWURST

1	egg	1
¹/₄ cup	cold milk	60 milliliters
¹/₄ teaspoon	caraway seeds	1 milliliter
1 teaspoon	parsley flakes	5 milliliters
¹/₄ teaspoon	ground coriander	1 milliliter
1 teaspoon	ground dry lemon peel	5 milliliters
¹/₄ teaspoon	ground mace	1 milliliter
¹/₄ teaspoon	ground mustard	1 milliliter
1 tablespoon	onion or leek (diced)	15 milliliters
1 tablespoon	onion powder	15 milliliters
¹/₄ teaspoon	paprika	1 milliliter
³/₄ teaspoon	ground white pepper	4 millilitres
1 teaspoon	salt	5 milliliters
¹/₄ teaspoon	brown sugar	1 milliliter
1 pound	freshly ground beef	500 grams
1 cup	uncooked oatmeal	250 milliliters

Combine egg and milk in a large bowl. Crush caraway seeds and parsley flakes in mortar with pestle. Blend all seasonings into the liquid. Add beef and oatmeal. Mix sausage the old-fashioned way, following directions on page 109. Make eight patties or links per recipe.

Yield: 8 servings
Exchange: (1 serving) 1 high-fat meat
Calories: (1 serving) 119

VEAL AND PORK BRATWURST

1	egg	1
¹/₄ cup	ice water	60 milliliters
³/₄ teaspoon	caraway seeds	4 milliliters
¹/₂ teaspoon	celery seeds	2 milliliters
¹/₄ teaspoon	allspice	1 milliliter
¹/₄ teaspoon	ground coriander	1 milliliter
³/₄ teaspoon	ground dry lemon peel	4 milliliters
¹/₄ teaspoon	ground nutmeg	1 milliliter
³/₄ teaspoon	onion powder or flakes	4 milliliters
¹/₂ teaspoon	parsely flakes	2 milliliters
³/₄ teaspoon	ground black pepper	4 milliliters
1 teaspoon	salt	5 milliliters
¹/₂ pound	freshly ground veal	250 grams
¹/₂ pound	freshly ground pork	250 grams
1 cup	Kellogg's All-Bran cereal	250 milliliters

In a large bowl, mix the egg and water. Crush caraway and celery seeds in a mortar with pestle. Blend seasonings into the liquid. Add veal, pork and cereal. Mix sausage the old-fashioned way, following directions on page 109. Make eight patties or links per recipe. Bratwurst should be refrigerated and used within a day or two.

Yield: 8 servings
Exchange: (1 serving) 2 medium-fat meat
Calories: (1 serving) 139

VIENNESE-STYLE SAUSAGE

¹/₂ cup	ice-cold milk	125 milliliters
1 tablespoon	all-purpose flour	15 milliliters
¹/₂ teaspoon	ground coriander	2 milliliters
¹/₄ teaspoon	ground mace	1 milliliter
1 tablespoon	onion (diced)	15 milliliters
¹/₂ teaspoon	ground paprika	2 milliliters
¹/₄ teaspoon	cayenne pepper	1 milliliter
1 teaspoon	salt	5 milliliters
¹/₄ teaspoon	sugar	1 milliliter
¹/₂ pound	freshly ground beef	250 grams
¹/₂ pound	freshly ground pork	250 grams
1 cup	white cornmeal	250 milliliters

Viennese-style sausage is delightful when smothered in hot tomato sauce and served as an appetizer or as the meat in your favorite casserole. Pour milk into a quart (liter) jar. Sprinkle flour into the jar, cover and shake to blend. Pour milk and flour solution into a large bowl. Blend seasonings into the liquid. Add beef, pork and cornmeal. Mix sausage the old-fashioned way, following directions on page 109.

Yield: 16 servings
Exchange: (1 serving) 1²/₃ high-fat meat
Calories: (1 serving) 173

Note: Add exchanges and calories for all other foods used with Viennese-style sausage.

PARISIENNE-STYLE SAUSAGE

¹/₂ **cup**	Burgundy wine (chilled)	125 milliliters
1 **tablespoon**	white flour	15 milliliters
¹/₄ **teaspoon**	ground bay leaf	1 milliliter
¹/₄ **teaspoon**	ground clove	1 milliliter
¹/₄ **teaspoon**	ground coriander	1 milliliter
¹/₄ **teaspoon**	ground ginger	1 milliliter
¹/₄ **teaspoon**	ground mace	1 milliliter
¹/₂ **teaspoon**	ground nutmeg	2 milliliters
1 **teaspoon**	ground black pepper	5 milliliters
1¹/₄ **teaspoons**	salt	6 milliliters
¹/₂ **teaspoon**	ground savory	2 milliliters
¹/₄ **teaspoon**	sugar	1 milliliter
¹/₄ **teaspoon**	ground tarragon	1 milliliter
¹/₄ **teaspoon**	ground thyme	1 milliliter
¹/₂ **pound**	freshly ground pork	250 grams
¹/₂ **pound**	freshly ground beef	250 grams
1 **cup**	yellow cornmeal	250 milliliters

Pour chilled wine into a large bowl. Blend flour and seasonings into the wine. Add pork, beef and cornmeal. Mix sausage the old-fashioned way, following directions on page 109.

Yield: 16 servings
Exchange: (1 serving) 1 medium-fat meat
Calories: (1 serving) 66

GREEK-STYLE LOUKANIKA

½ cup	rosé wine (chilled)	125 milliliters
2 tablespoons	orange juice (chilled)	30 milliliters
¼ teaspoon	ground allspice	1 milliliter
¼ teaspoon	ground cinnamon	1 milliliter
¼ teaspoon	ground cumin	1 milliliter
1 clove	garlic (minced)	1 clove
¼ teaspoon	ground nutmeg	1 milliliter
2 tablespoons	orange peel (grated)	30 milliliters
¼ teaspoon	ground black pepper	1 milliliter
½ teaspoon	peppercorns (cracked)	2 milliliters
1 teaspoon	salt	5 milliliters
1 teaspoon	dried savory	5 milliliters
¼ teaspoon	brown sugar	1 milliliter
½ pound	freshly ground veal	250 grams
½ pound	freshly ground pork	250 grams
1 cup	bulgur	250 milliliters

Loukanika can be served as a main dish for dinner or on Greek-style bread as a luncheon meal. Mix wine and orange juice in a large bowl. Blend all seasonings into the liquid. Add veal, pork and bulgur. Mix sausage the old-fashioned way, following directions on page 109. Make 8 patties or links per recipe.

Yield: 8 servings
Exchange: (1 serving) 2 medium-fat meat
Calories: (1 serving) 139

Note: Add exchanges and calories for all other foods used with loukanika.

ITALIAN-STYLE SAUSAGE

Italian sausage is a worldwide favorite. Sweet or hot Italian sausage can be served as a main dish, on a slice of hot Italian bread, as the meat sauce on spaghetti or as a pizza topping. Use your imagination to create delightful menus using the following delicious sausages.

SWEET ITALIAN-STYLE SAUSAGE

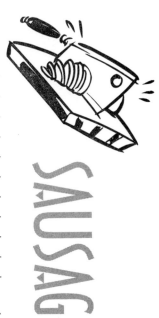

1/2 cup	ice water	125 milliliters
3/4 teaspoon	aniseed	4 milliliters
1/2 teaspoon	ground coriander	2 milliliters
1/2 teaspoon	ground paprika	2 milliliters
1/4 teaspoon	ground black pepper	1 milliliter
1/4 teaspoon	ground cayenne pepper	1 milliliter
1/4 teaspoon	cayenne pepper flakes	1 milliliter
3/4 teaspoon	salt	4 milliliters
1/4 teaspoon	brown sugar	1 milliliter
1 pound	freshly ground pork	500 grams
1 cup	bulgur	250 milliliters

Pour ice water into a large bowl. Crush aniseed with mortar and pestle. Blend seasonings into the liquid. Add pork and bulgur. Mix sausage the old-fashioned way, following directions on page 109. Make 8 patties or links per recipe.

Yield: 8 servings
Exchange: (1 serving) 1 1/2 high-fat meat
Calories: (1 serving) 156

HOT ITALIAN-STYLE SAUSAGE

1/2 cup	dry Italian red wine	125 milliliters
1/2 teaspoon	fennel seed	2 milliliters
1 teaspoon	liquid smoke	5 milliliters
1 teaspoon	paprika	5 milliliters
1 teaspoon	cayenne pepper	5 milliliters
3/4 teaspoon	cayenne pepper flakes	4 milliliters
1 teaspoon	salt	5 milliliters
1 pound	freshly ground pork	500 grams
1 cup	40% bran flakes	250 milliliters

Chill the wine. Pour into a large bowl. Crush fennel seed with mortar and pestle. Blend all seasonings into the liquid. Add pork and 40% bran flakes. Mix sausage the old-fashioned way, following directions on page 109. Make 8 patties or links per recipe.

Yield: 8 servings
Exchange: (1 serving) 2 medium-fat meat
Calories: (1 serving) 151

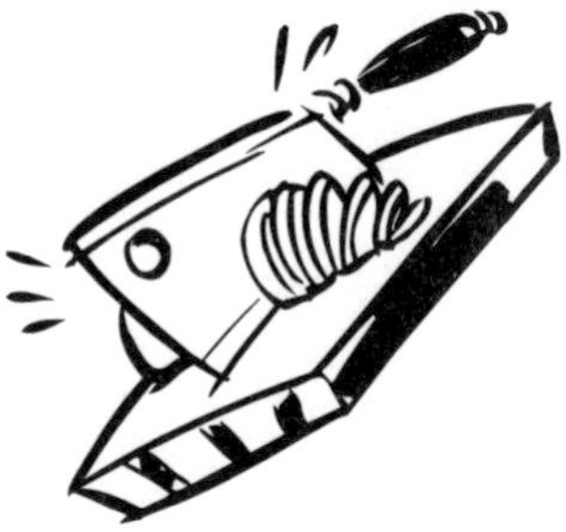

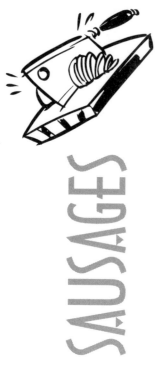

LUGANEGA—NORTHERN ITALIAN-STYLE SAUSAGE

1/2 cup	Italian white vermouth	125 milliliters
2 tablespoons	orange juice	30 milliliters
4 tablespoons	Parmesan cheese (grated)	45 milliliters
1/4 teaspoon	ground coriander	1 milliliter
1 clove	garlic (minced)	1 clove
1/4 teaspoon	ground dry lemon peel	1 milliliter
1/4 teaspoon	ground nutmeg	1 milliliter
1/4 teaspoon	ground dry orange peel	1 milliliter
1/4 teaspoon	ground black pepper	1 milliliter
3/4 teaspoon	salt	4 milliliters
1 pound	freshly ground pork	500 grams
1 cup	wheat germ	250 milliliters

Chill vermouth and pour into a large bowl. Blend seasonings into the liquid. Add pork and wheat germ. Mix sausage the old-fashioned way, following directions on page 109. Make 8 patties or links per recipe.

Yield: 8 servings
Exchange: (1 serving) 2 high-fat meat
Calories: (1 serving) 188

Note: Add exchanges and calories for all other foods used with loukanika.

NEAR EASTERN-STYLE SAUSAGE

1/2 cup	ice water	125 milliliters
dash	ground allspice	dash
1/4 teaspoon	ground cloves	1 milliliter
2 cloves	garlic (minced)	2 cloves
1/4 teaspoon	ground oregano	1 milliliter
1/2 teaspoon	ground black pepper	2 milliliters
1/2 teaspoon	ground rosemary	2 milliliters
1 teaspoon	salt	5 milliliters
1/4 teaspoon	sugar	1 milliliter
1 pound	freshly ground lamb	500 grams
1 cup	bran flakes	250 milliliters

Serve as a main dish, baked with your favorite casserole or on pita bread with condiments. Pour ice water into a large bowl. Blend seasonings into the liquid. Add lamb and bran flakes. Mix sausage the old-fashioned way, following directions on page 109. Make 8 patties or links per recipe.

> **Yield:** 8 servings
> **Exchange:** (1 serving) 1 high-fat meat or 2 lean meat
> **Calories:** (1 serving) 118

Note: Add calories and exchanges for condiments or other foods served with Near Eastern-style sausage.

POLISH-STYLE SAUSAGE

Polish-style sausage, a favorite throughout the Western World, can be served on a whole wheat or rye bun with your favorite condiments. This sausage is great as a main dish all by itself or cooked with sauerkraut. You can be creative and develop your own favorite menus featuring Polish-style sausage.

MILD POLISH-STYLE SAUSAGE

1/2 **cup**	ice water	125 milliliters
1/4 **teaspoon**	celery seed	1 milliliter
1/2 **teaspoon**	garlic powder	2 milliliters
1/2 **teaspoon**	ground marjoram	2 milliliters
dash	ground or grated nutmeg	dash
1/2 **teaspoon**	ground black pepper	2 milliliters
1 **teaspoon**	salt	5 milliliters
1/4 **teaspoon**	brown sugar	1 milliliter
1/4 **teaspoon**	ground thyme	1 milliliter
1/2 **pound**	freshly ground beef	250 grams
1/2 **pound**	freshly ground pork	250 grams
1 **cup**	40% bran flakes	250 milliliters

Pour water into a large bowl. Blend seasonings into the liquid. Add beef, pork and bran flakes. Mix sausage the old-fashioned way, following directions on page 109. Make 8 patties or links per recipe.

> **Yield:** 8 servings
> **Exchange:** (1 serving) 2 medium-fat meat
> **Calories:** (1 serving) 122

SPICY POLISH-STYLE SAUSAGE

1/2 **cup**	ice-cold beer	125 milliliters
1 teaspoon	liquid smoke	5 milliliters
1/4 **teaspoon**	ground allspice	1 milliliter
1/2 **teaspoon**	celery seed	2 milliliters
1/4 **teaspoon**	ground coriander	1 milliliter
2 cloves	garlic (minced)	2 cloves
1/2 **teaspoon**	ground marjoram	2 milliliters
1/4 **teaspoon**	ground mace	1 milliliter
1 teaspoon	ground paprika	5 milliliters
1 teaspoon	ground white pepper	5 milliliters
3/4 **teaspoon**	salt	4 milliliters
1/2 **teaspoon**	ground thyme	2 milliliters
1/4 **pound**	freshly ground beef	125 grams
3/4 **pound**	freshly ground pork	375 grams
1 cup	bulgur	250 milliliters

Pour beer into a large bowl. Blend seasonings into the beer. Add beef, pork, and bulgur. Mix sausage the old-fashioned way, following directions on page 109. Make 8 patties or links per recipe.

Yield: 8 servings
Exchange: (1 serving) 1 1/2 high-fat meat
Calories: (1 serving) 147

RUSSIAN-STYLE KIELBASA

1/2 **cup**	ice water	125 milliliters
1 teaspoon	vinegar	5 milliliters
1/4 **teaspoon**	dillseed	1 milliliter
1/4 **teaspoon**	ground allspice	1 milliliter
1/4 **teaspoon**	celery flakes	1 milliliter
1/4 **teaspoon**	cinnamon	1 milliliter
2 cloves	garlic (minced)	2 cloves
1/2 **teaspoon**	ground marjoram	2 milliliters
1/4 **teaspoon**	paprika	1 milliliter
1 teaspoon	ground black pepper	5 milliliters
3/4 **teaspoon**	salt	4 milliliters
1 pound	freshly ground beef	500 grams
1/2 **cup**	oatmeal	125 milliliters
1/2 **cup**	wheat germ	125 milliliters

Combine water and vinegar in a large bowl. Crack dillseed in a mortar and pestle. Blend seasonings into the liquid. Add beef, oatmeal, and wheat germ. Mix sausage the old-fashioned way, following directions on page 109. Make 8 patties or links per recipe.

Yield: 8 servings
Exchange: (1 serving) 1¼ high-fat meat
Calories: (1 serving) 126

Note: Add calories and exchanges for condiments or other foods served with Russian-style kielbasa.

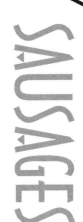

SCANDINAVIAN-STYLE POTATO SAUSAGE

¼ **cup**	ice-cold milk	60 milliliters
1	egg	1
¼ **teaspoon**	allspice	1 milliliter
dash	ground mace	dash
¼ **teaspoon**	ground nutmeg	1 milliliter
4 tablespoons	onion (minced)	60 milliliters
1 teaspoon	ground black pepper	5 milliliters
1 teaspoon	salt	5 milliliters
¼ **teaspoon**	brown sugar	1 milliliter
½ **pound**	freshly ground beef	250 grams
½ **pound**	freshly ground pork	250 grams
½ **cup**	bran flakes	125 milliliters
½ **cup**	dried instant potatoes	125 milliliters

Combine egg and milk in a large bowl. Blend seasonings into the liquid. Add beef, pork, bran flakes and potatoes. Mix sausage the old-fashioned way, following directions on page 109. Make 8 patties or links per recipe.

Yield: 8 servings
Exchange: (1 serving) 1½ high-fat meat or 2 medium-fat meat
Calories: (1 serving) 143

SPANISH-STYLE CHORIZO

Chorizo is prized throughout the Spanish-speaking world. Serve spicy or hot chorizo as a main dish on a slice of hot bread or as the meat in a Spanish or Mexican dish. Use your imagination to create delightful menus using chorizo.

SAUSAGES

SPICY SPANISH-STYLE CHORIZO

¹/₂ **cup**	ice water	125 milliliters
1 tablespoon	cider vinegar	15 milliliters
¹/₂ **teaspoon**	aniseed	2 milliliters
¹/₄ **teaspoon**	chili powder	1 milliliter
¹/₄ **teaspoon**	ground cumin	1 milliliter
¹/₂ **teaspoon**	garlic powder	2 milliliters
1 teaspoon	ground marjoram	5 milliliters
2 tablespoons	onion (minced)	30 milliliters
¹/₂ **teaspoon**	ground paprika	2 milliliters
¹/₄ **teaspoon**	ground black pepper	1 milliliter
¹/₂ **teaspoon**	cayenne pepper	2 milliliters
¹/₂ **teaspoon**	cayenne pepper flakes	2 milliliters
1 teaspoon	salt	5 milliliters
¹/₄ **teaspoon**	brown sugar	1 milliliter
1 pound	freshly ground pork	500 grams
1 cup	yellow cornmeal	250 milliliters

Combine water and vinegar in a large bowl. Crush aniseed with mortar and pestle. Blend seasonings into the liquid. Add pork and cornmeal. Mix sausage the old-fashioned way, following directions on page 109. Make 8 patties or links per recipe.

Yield: 8 servings
Exchange: (1 serving) 2 high-fat meat
Calories: (1 serving) 180

HOT SPANISH-STYLE CHORIZO

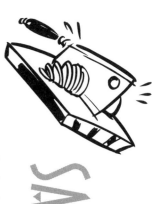

¹/₂ **cup**	red wine (chilled)	125 milliliters
1 tablespoon	cider vinegar	15 milliliters
1 teaspoon	dark corn syrup	5 milliliters
¹/₂ **teaspoon**	fennel seed	2 milliliters
1 teaspoon	chili powder	5 milliliters
¹/₂ **teaspoon**	ground cumin	2 milliliters
2 cloves	garlic (minced)	2 cloves
1 tablespoon	onion powder	15 milliliters
1 teaspoon	ground oregano	5 milliliters
2 teaspoons	ground paprika	10 milliliters
1 teaspoon	cayenne pepper	5 milliliters
1 teaspoon	cayenne pepper flakes	5 milliliters
³/₄ **teaspoon**	salt	4 milliliters
1 pound	freshly ground pork	500 grams
1 cup	wheat germ	250 millilitres

Mix wine, vinegar and corn syrup in a large mixing bowl. Crush fennel seed in mortar with pestle. Blend seasonings into the liquid. Add pork and wheat germ. Mix sausage the old-fashioned way, following directions on page 109. Make 8 patties or links per recipe.

Yield:	8 servings
Exchange:	(1 serving) 2 high-fat meat
Calories:	(1 serving) 196

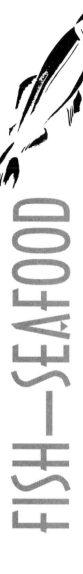

FISH—SEAFOOD

FISH FLORENTINE

2 tablespoons	onion (chopped)	30 milliliters
¹/₂ cup	mushrooms (chopped)	125 milliliters
1 tablespoon	margarine	15 milliliters
2 cups	cooked spinach (well drained)	500 milliliters
1 teaspoon	lemon juice	5 milliliters
1 cup	White Sauce (page 164)	250 milliliters
3 ounces	Cheddar cheese (grated)	90 grams
12 ounces	cooked fish (flaked)	360 grams

Sauté onion and mushrooms in margarine until onion is transparent. Add spinach and lemon juice; mix well. Pour into baking dish or 6 individual baking dishes coated with vegetable cooking spray. Cover with ¹/₂ cup (125 milliliters) of the White Sauce. Sprinkle with 1¹/₂ ounces (45 milliliters) of the cheese. Cover with fish, then with remaining sauce. Sprinkle with remaining cheese. Bake at 350°F (175°C) for 20 minutes.

Microwave: Cook on MEDIUM for 10 minutes; turn. Cook 5 minutes more. Hold 3 minutes.

> **Yield:** 6 servings
> **Exchange:** (1 serving) 3¹/₂ high-fat meat, 1 vegetable, 1 bread, ¹/₂ milk, 1 fat
> **Calories:** (1 serving) 215

BROILED TROUT

5 ounces	trout fillet	150 grams
1 teaspoon	margarine	5 milliliters
dash each	lemon, pepper, marjoram, salt, paprika	dash each

Clean trout fillet thoroughly; pat dry. Melt margarine; brush on both sides of fillet. Sprinkle with seasonings in order given. Broil 5 to 6 inches (12 to 15 centimeters) from heat for 10 to 15 minutes. It is not necessary to turn the fillet.

> **Yield:** 1 serving
> **Exchange:** 5 lean meat, 1 fat
> **Calories:** 190

POACHED FISH

2 pounds	fish (haddock, cod, pollack, salmon)	1 kilogram
1 quart	water	1 liter
1	carrot (sliced)	1
1	onion (sliced)	1
1	bay leaf	1
¹/₂ teaspoon	thyme	2 milliliters
¹/₂ teaspoon	whole peppercorns	2 milliliters

Wash fish; wrap in cheesecloth. Combine remaining ingredients in large kettle. Bring to a boil; reduce heat and cook for 15 minutes. Add fish and cook at a simmer. Time depends on thickness, not weight; cook 10 minutes for each inch (2.5 centimeters) of thickness. Drain in cheesecloth. Turn out onto warm serving platter. Remove skin carefully.

Note: Yield is not listed for some recipes where some people are allowed 1 exchange while others are allowed 2 or more.

Exchange: (1 ounce/30 grams) 1 meat
Calories: (1 ounce/30 grams) 21

Note: Bone is not counted in serving weight.

BROILED SMELT

3 ounces	smelt	90 grams
	salt & pepper to taste	
1 teaspoon	margarine	5 milliliters
1 teaspoon	lemon juice	5 milliliters

Dry smelt thoroughly. Salt and pepper cavity of smelt. Melt margarine; brush on both sides of smelt. Sprinkle with lemon juice. Add salt and pepper. Broil 6 to 8 inches (15 to 20 centimeters) from heat for 10 to 15 minutes.

Yield: 1 serving
Exchange: 3 medium-fat meat
Calories: 95

FISH—SEAFOOD

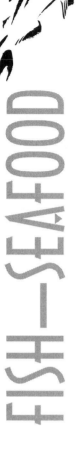

BAKED WHITEFISH

1 teaspoon	margarine	5 milliliters
3 ounces	whitefish fillet	90 grams
	salt & pepper to taste	

Melt margarine; brush on both sides of fish fillet. Place fish on aluminum foil. Add salt and pepper. Wrap tightly, securing ends. Place on baking sheet. Bake at 375°F (190°C) for 45 minutes.

Microwave: Wrap in plastic; prick wrap. Place on cooking rack. Cook for 7 to 8 minutes, giving package a quarter turn after 4 minutes.

      Yield: 1 serving
Exchange: 3 medium-fat meat, 1 fat
  Calories: 229

MUSTARD HALIBUT STEAKS

3 ounces	halibut steak	90 grams
1 teaspoon	margarine	5 milliliters
1 teaspoon	lemon juice	5 milliliters
1/2 teaspoon	Dijon mustard	2 milliliters
dash each	lemon rind, sugar replacement	dash each
	salt to taste	

Wash and dry halibut thoroughly. Melt margarine; brush on both sides of halibut. Lay on broiler pan. Brush top with mixture of lemon juice, Dijon mustard and seasonings. Broil 5 to 6 inches (12 to 15 centimeters) from heat for 3 to 4 minutes. Turn halibut; repeat on second side.

      Yield: 1 serving
Exchange: 1 lean meat, 1 fat
  Calories: 90

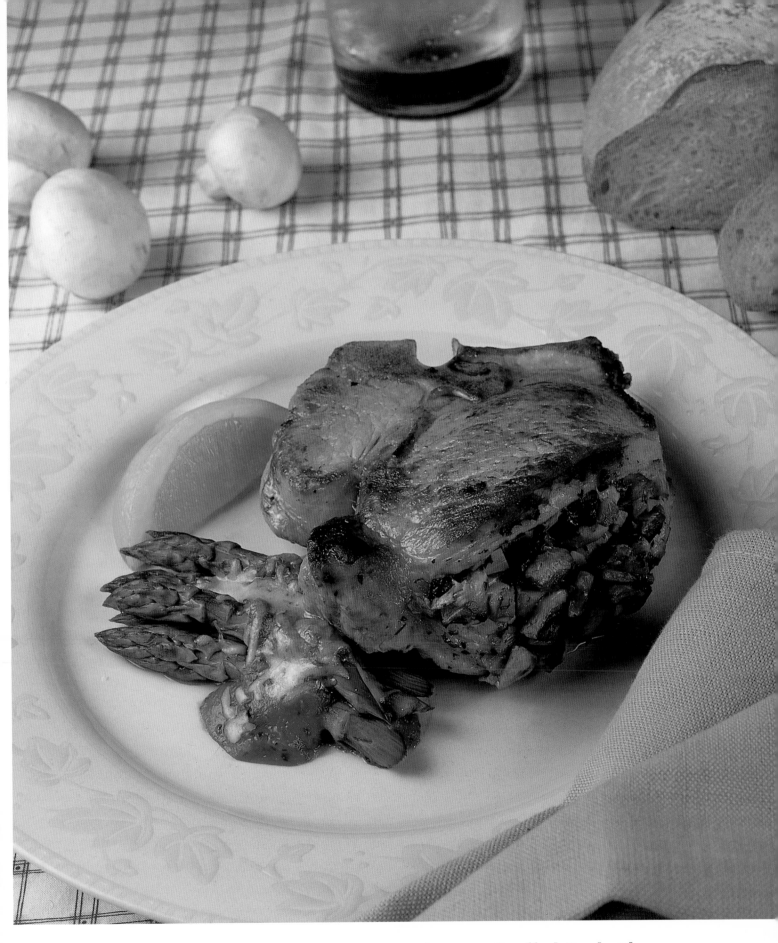

Italian Asparagus

•••

see page 153

& Mushroom-Stuffed Pork Chops

•••

see page 98

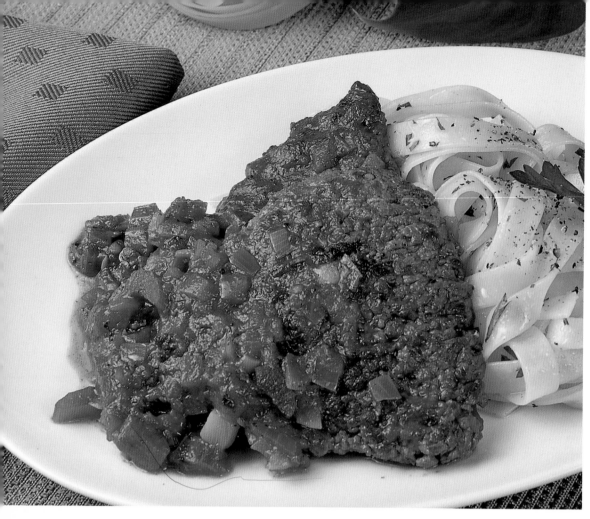

Swiss Steak
• • •
see page 105

**Greek-Style
Loukanika**
• • •
see page 118

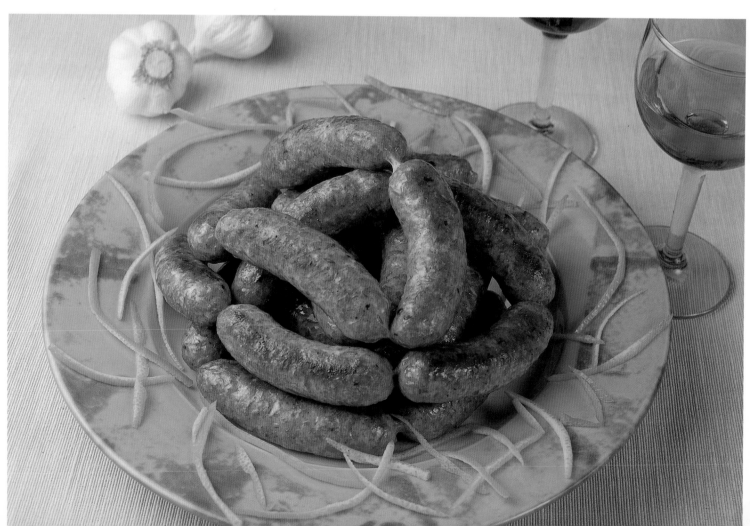

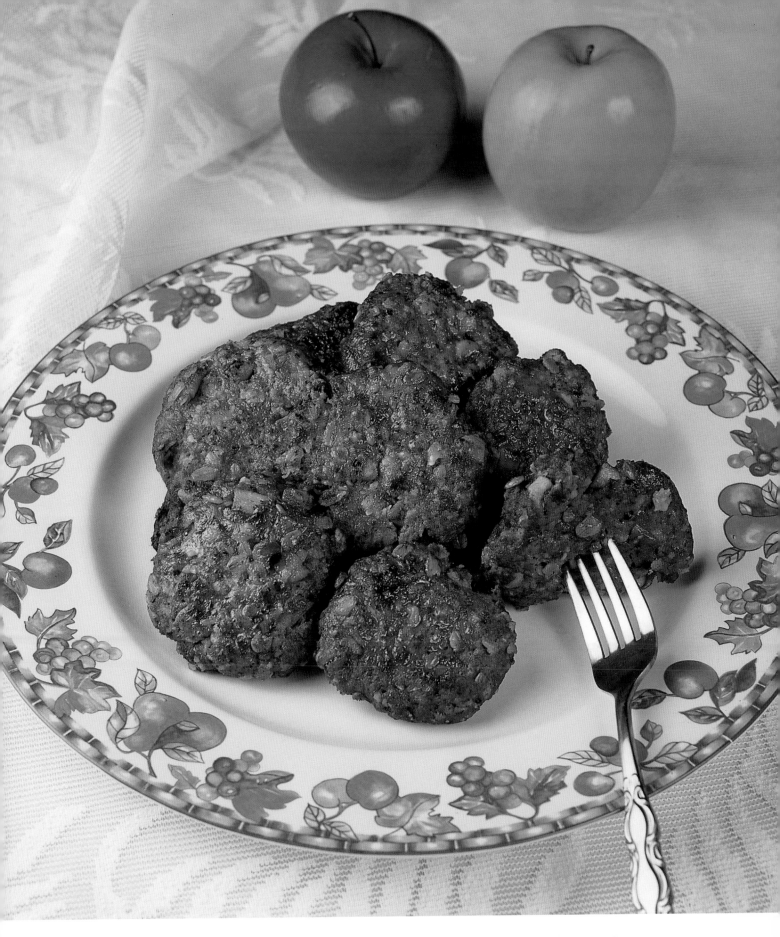

Sweet Beef with Apples Breakfast Sausage

• • •

see page 110

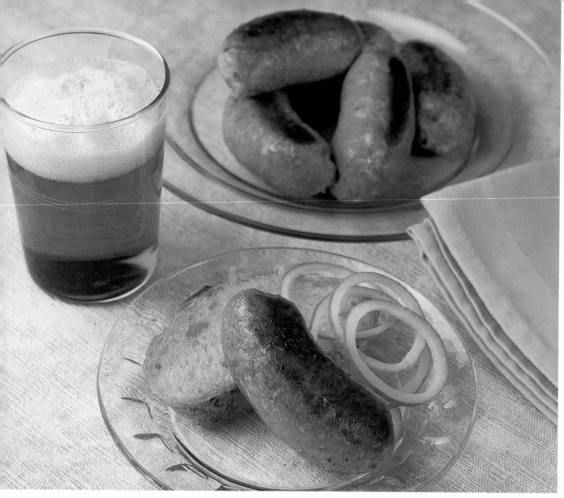

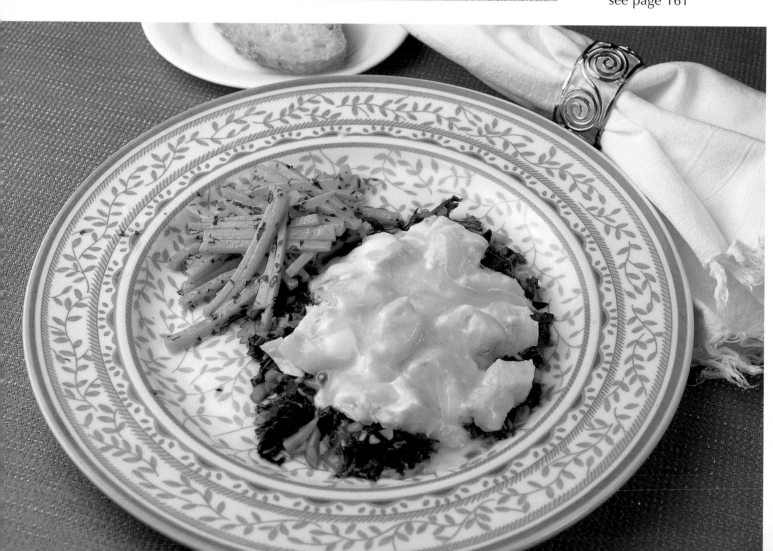

Spicy Spanish-Style Chorizo
• • •
see page 124

Fish Florentine
see page 126
• • •
& Circus Carrots
see page 161

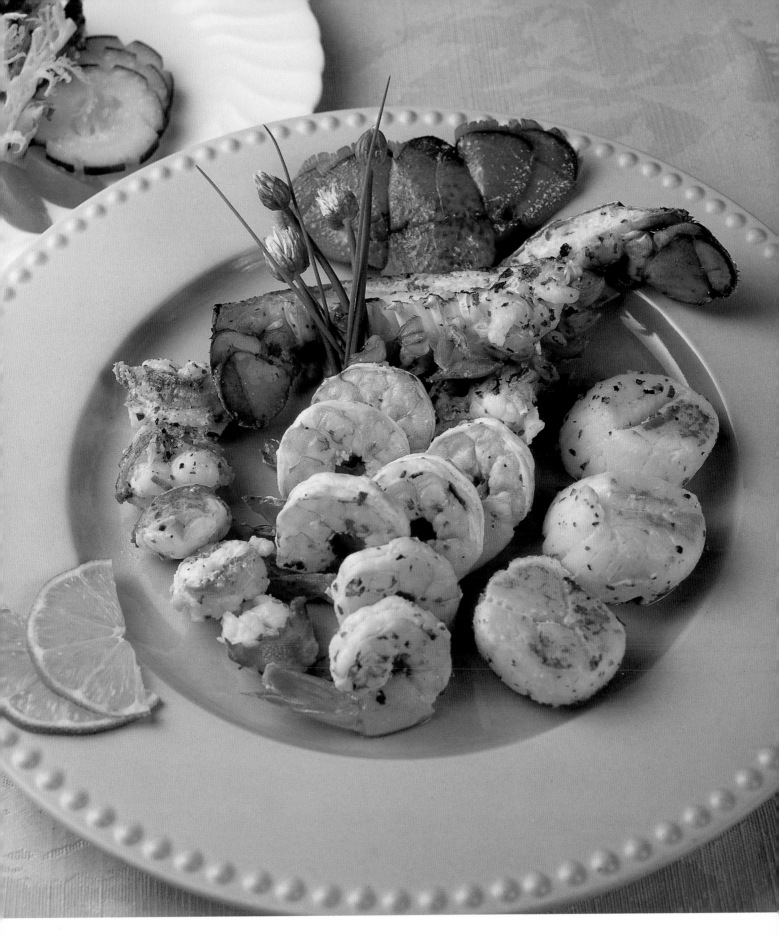

Venetian Seafood

• • •

see page 134

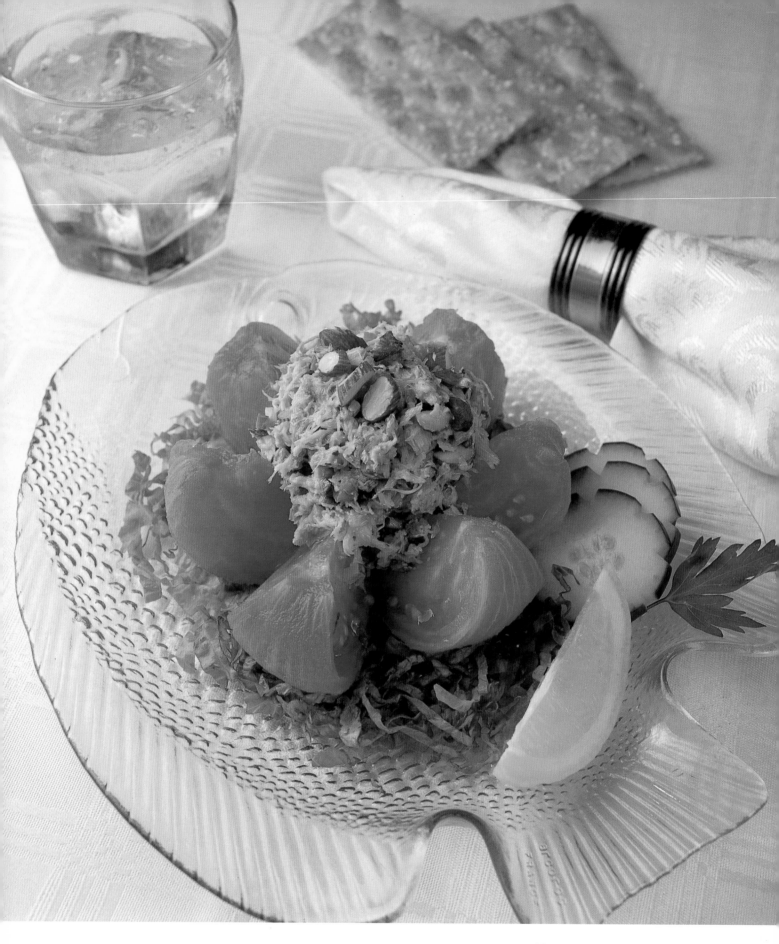

Tomato Stuffed with Crab Louis

• • •

see page 135

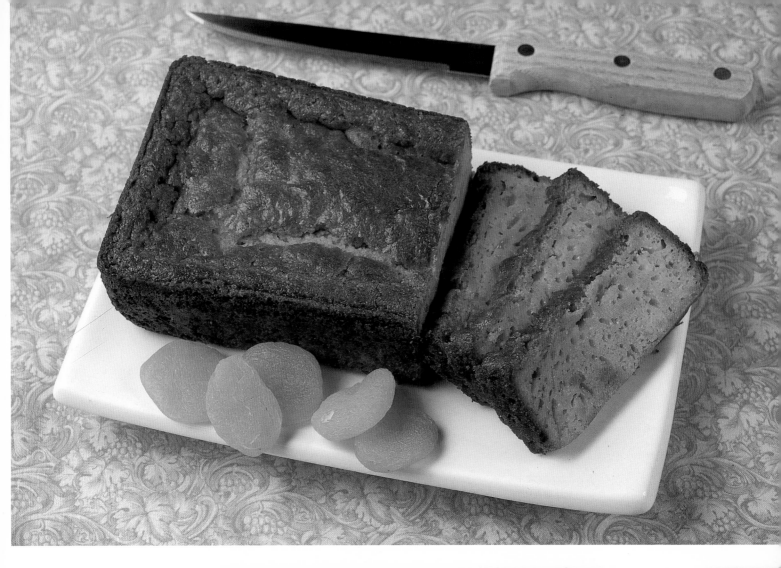

Apricot Bread

• • •

see page 139

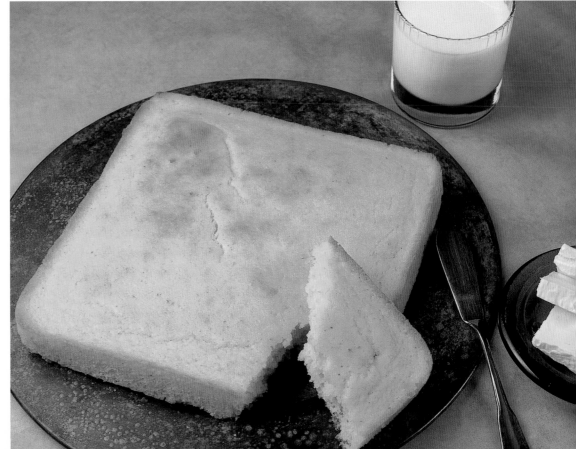

Pioneer Cornbread

• • •

see page 141

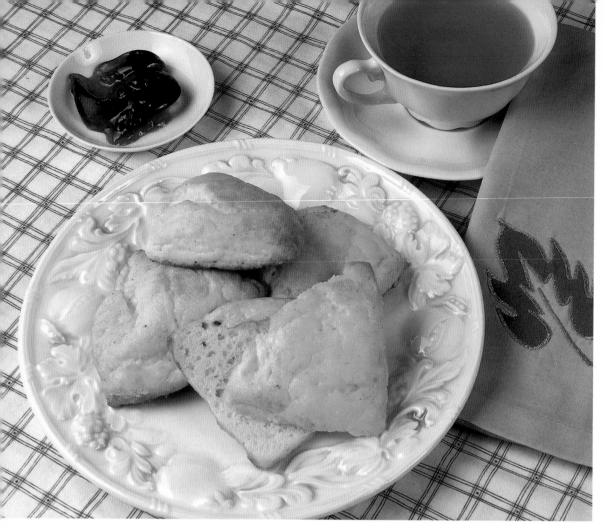

Tea Scones

• • •

see page 144

ABC's of Vegetables

• • •

see page 151

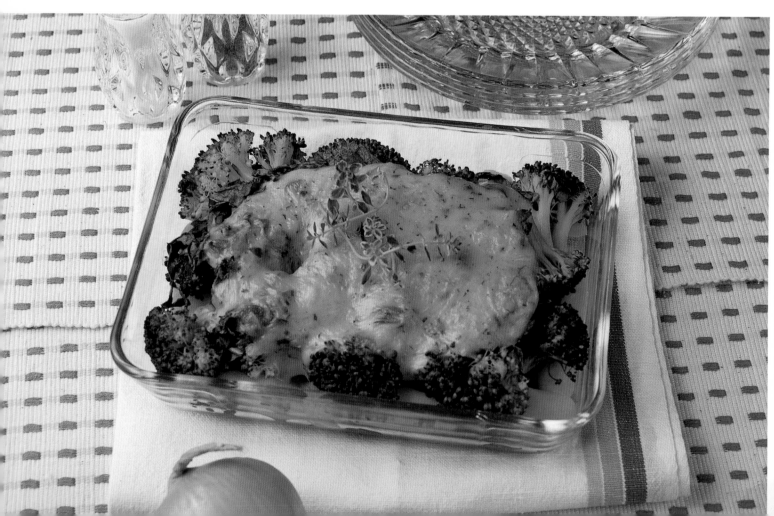

FISH CREOLE

2 pounds	whitefish fillets	1 kilogram
3 cups	water	750 milliliters
1	bay leaf	1
3 stalks	celery with tops (chopped)	3 stalks
	salt & pepper to taste	
2 cups	Creole Sauce (page 165)	500 milliliters

Cut fish into serving pieces. Combine water, bay leaf, celery, salt, and pepper in saucepan. Boil for 2 to 3 minutes. Remove from heat. Add fish pieces and allow water to cool completely. Drain fish and celery; remove bay leaf. Heat Creole sauce. Add fish and celery. Simmer on low heat for 5 minutes.

Yield: 6 servings
Exchange: (1 serving) 5 medium-fat meat
Calories: (1 serving) 370

INDIVIDUAL MACKEREL

3 ounces	cooked mackerel (flaked)	90 grams
2 tablespoons	mushrooms (chopped)	30 milliliters
1 teaspoon	onion (finely chopped)	5 milliliters
1 teaspoon	celery (finely chopped)	5 milliliters
1/2 slice	bread (crumbled)	1/2 slice
1/2 teaspoon	parsley (finely chopped)	2 milliliters
1	egg (beaten)	1
1 teaspoon	ketchup	5 milliliters
	salt & pepper to taste	

Combine all ingredients. Mix thoroughly. Place in small baking dish. Bake at 350°F (175°C) for 40 minutes.

Microwave: Cook on MEDIUM for 10 to 12 minutes.

Yield: 1 serving
Exchange: 4 medium-fat meat, 1/2 bread
Calories: 322

FISH—SEAFOOD

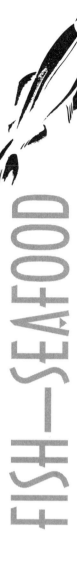

SALMON LOAF

16 ounces	cooked salmon (flaked)	500 grams
2 tablespoons	onion (chopped)	30 milliliters
3 tablespoons	vegetable juice	45 milliliters
¼ teaspoon	marjoram	1 milliliter
2	eggs	2
1 cup	bread crumbs (finely ground)	250 milliliters
	salt & pepper to taste	

If canned salmon is used, drain thoroughly. Combine with remaining ingredients. Blend thoroughly. Allow to rest for 5 minutes, or until bread crumbs are soft. Blend again. Line a 9 x 5-inch (23 x 13-centimeter) loaf pan with waxed paper. Pack salmon mixture tightly into loaf pan. Bake at 350°F (175°C) for 40 minutes.

Yield: 6 servings
Exchange: (1 serving) 3 medium-fat meat, ½ bread
Calories: (1 serving) 255

FINNAN HADDIE

3 ounces	cooked finnan haddie	90 grams
1 tablespoon	leek (chopped)	15 milliliters
1 tablespoon	green pepper (chopped)	15 milliliters
2 teaspoons	pimientos (chopped)	10 milliliters
¼ cup	condensed cream of mushroom soup	60 milliliters
½ ounce	Cheddar cheese (grated)	15 grams
	salt & pepper to taste	

Arrange finnan haddie in baking dish. Combine leek, green pepper, pimientos, and condensed soup. Stir to mix. Add salt and pepper. Pour over fish. Top with cheese. Bake at 350°F (175°C) for 20 to 25 minutes.

Microwave: Cook on MEDIUM for 10 minutes. Turn once.

Yield: 1 serving
Exchange: 3½ medium-fat meat, ½ bread, 1 fat
Calories: 220

BAKED TURBOT

4 ounces	turbot fillet	120 grams
1 teaspoon	margarine	5 milliliters
1 teaspoon	lemon juice	5 milliliters
dash each	salt, pepper, paprika, parsley	dash each

Clean turbot fillet thoroughly; pat dry. Melt margarine; brush on both sides of fillet. Place on aluminum foil. Sprinkle with lemon juice, then seasonings. Wrap up fillet securely; lay in cake pan. Bake at 350°F (175°C) for 30 to 40 minutes. Slide fish out of foil onto warm serving plate.

Yield: 1 serving
Exchange: 4 medium-fat meat, 1 fat
Calories: 400

COOKED FLAKED FISH

1 pound	any raw fish	500 grams

Clean fish and cook in salted boiling water for 15 to 20 minutes. Remove skin and bones. Flake fish.

Exchange: (1 ounce/30 grams) 1 meat
Calories: (1 ounce/30 grams) 25

GREAT CRAB

2 ounces	crabmeat	60 grams
1 teaspoon	butter	5 milliliters
dash each	lemon juice, parsley, rosemary, salt, paprika	dash each

Melt butter in small saucepan. Mix in lemon juice and seasonings. Add crabmeat. Toss to coat and heat.

Yield: 1 serving
Exchange: 2 lean meat, 1 fat
Calories: 100

FISH—SEAFOOD

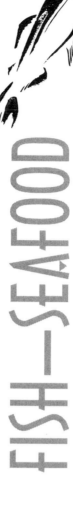

MARINATED CRAB LEGS

¹/₂ cup	Teriyaki Marinade (page 165)	125 milliliters
¹/₃ cup	lemon juice	80 milliliters
¹/₂ cup	water	125 milliliters
1 teaspoon	basil	5 milliliters
1 to 2 pounds	cooked crab legs (shelled)	500 to 1000 grams

Combine marinade, lemon juice, water, and basil. Add crab legs. (If necessary, add more water to cover legs.) Marinate 2 to 3 hours.

Exchange: (1 ounce/30 grams) 1 lean meat
Calories: (1 ounce/30 grams) 32

OYSTERS ON THE SHELL

2 ounces	oysters	60 grams
2 tablespoons	mushroom pieces	30 milliliters
1 teaspoon	onion (diced)	5 milliliters
¹/₄ cup	vegetable broth	60 milliliters
1 slice	bread (finely crumbled)	1 slice
¹/₄ teaspoon	lemon juice	1 milliliter
1	oyster shell	1
¹/₄ ounce	Cheddar cheese (grated)	8 grams
	salt & pepper to taste	

Cook oysters in small amount of boiling salted water until edges start to curl. Drain (reserve some liquid). Combine mushrooms, onion, and broth in saucepan. Bring to a boil. Reduce heat. Add bread crumbs; stir to mix. Remove from heat. Add lemon juice and enough reserved oyster liquid to moisten bread-crumb mixture thoroughly. Add oysters, salt, and pepper. Heap into shell or small baking dish. Top with cheese. Broil until cheese melts.

Yield: 1 serving
Exchange: 2¹/₂ lean meat, 1 bread
Calories: 125

CLAM MOUSSE

1 packet	unflavored gelatin	1 packet
1 cube	vegetable bouillon	1 cube
1/2 cup	boiling water	125 millilitres
8 ounces	minced clams (& juice)	240 grams
8 ounces	yogurt	240 grams
1 teaspoon	lemon juice	5 millilitres
1 teaspoon	celery flakes	5 millilitres
1 teaspoon	parsley flakes	5 millilitres
	small dash cayenne	

Dissolve gelatin and bouillon cube in boiling water. Beat in remaining ingredients with whisk or electric mixer. Pour into mold and chill until firm.

       Yield: 4 servings
Exchange: (1 serving) 2 lean meat, 1/4 milk
  Calories: (1 serving) 70

SHRIMP SOUFFLÉ

2 ounces	shrimp (canned)	60 grams
dash each	thyme, rosemary (crushed), salt, pepper	dash each
1	egg (separated)	1
	vegetable cooking spray	

Break shrimp into fine pieces. Add to beaten egg yolk and seasonings. Beat egg whites until stiff. Gently stir half of egg white into shrimp mixture. Gently fold in remaining egg white. Pour into large individual soufflé dish coated with vegetable cooking spray. (Dish should be less than two-thirds full.) Bake at 375°F (190°C) for 15 to 20 minutes.

       Yield: 1 serving
Exchange: 3 lean meat
  Calories: 205

FISH—SEAFOOD

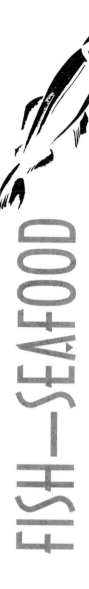

VENETIAN SEAFOOD

¹/₂ cup	water	125 milliliters
2 tablespoons	lime juice	30 milliliters
1 tablespoon	chives (finely chopped)	15 milliliters
1 teaspoon	garlic powder	5 milliliters
¹/₂ teaspoon	oregano	2 milliliters
¹/₂ teaspoon	salt	2 milliliters
¹/₄ teaspoon	pepper	1 milliliter
1 ounce	fresh or frozen lobster (thawed & cubed)	30 grams
1 ounce	fresh or frozen scallops (thawed)	30 grams
1 ounce	fresh or frozen shrimp (thawed)	30 grams
	vegetable cooking spray	

Make a marinade by blending water, lime juice, and seasonings. Place thawed seafood in deep narrow dish. Pour marinade over seafood to cover. Refrigerate for 3 to 5 hours. (Stir occasionally if seafood is not completely covered with marinade.) Drain. Spray seafood with vegetable cooking spray. Place on baking sheet or dish coated with vegetable cooking spray. Broil 5 to 6 inches (12 to 15 centimeters) from heat for 5 to 6 minutes until seafood is tender. Shake baking sheet or dish occasionally to brown seafood evenly.

Yield: 1 serving
Exchange: 3 lean meat
Calories: 90

SHRIMP CREOLE

¹/₂ cup	Creole Sauce (page 165)	125 milliliters
10	small shrimp	10
1 cup	rice (cooked)	250 milliliters

Heat Creole sauce just to a boil. Add shrimp. Remove from heat. Allow to rest 10 minutes. Serve over rice.

Yield: 1 serving
Exchange: 2 meat, 2 bread, ¹/₂ vegetable, 1 fat
Calories: 238

TOMATO STUFFED WITH CRAB LOUIS

1/2 teaspoon	ketchup	2 milliliters
1 teaspoon	mayonnaise	5 milliliters
1/4 teaspoon	Worcestershire sauce	1 milliliter
1 ounce	crabmeat	30 grams
1 teaspoon	green onion (finely chopped)	5 milliliters
1 tablespoon	celery (finely chopped)	15 milliliters
1 tablespoon	green pepper (finely chopped)	15 milliliters
1 teaspoon	parsley (finely chopped)	5 milliliters
3	almonds (chopped)	3
1	tomato (peeled)	1
1	lettuce leaf	1

To make Crab Louis, blend ketchup, mayonnaise, and Worcestershire sauce; add crabmeat, green onion, celery, green pepper, parsley, and almonds. Stir to bind; chill. Cut peeled tomato into 6 sections, slicing almost to the bottom. Fill with Crab Louis. Serve on lettuce leaf.

Yield: 1 serving
Exchange: 1 medium-fat meat, 1 fat, 1 vegetable
Calories: 110

LONG ISLAND BOIL

1 ounce	mussels	30 grams
1	tomato (peeled & quartered)	1
1	onion (cut into large chunks)	1
1/2 teaspoon	garlic powder	2 milliliters
1 teaspoon	parsley	5 milliliters
1 ounce	halibut (cut into chunks)	30 grams
1 ounce	scallops	30 grams
	salt & pepper to taste	

Wash mussels thoroughly. Soak in cold water overnight. Steam mussels until shells open; remove mussels from shells. Combine tomato, onion, garlic powder, and parsley. Simmer for 15 minutes. Add halibut and scallops. Cover; simmer 10 minutes. Add mussels, salt and pepper. Heat thoroughly.

Yield: 1 serving
Exchange: 3 lean meat, 1 vegetable
Calories: 105

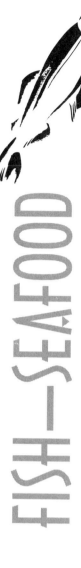

LOBSTER ORIENTALE

1 cup	chicken broth	250 milliliters
4	shallots	4
¹/₄ teaspoon	ginger	1 milliliter
¹/₄ teaspoon	curry powder	1 milliliter
1 ounce	pork (cubed)	30 grams
2 ounces	lobster (cubed)	60 grams
1 teaspoon	cornstarch	5 milliliters
¹/₄ cup	cold water	60 milliliters
¹/₂ cup	bean sprouts	125 milliliters

Combine chicken broth, shallots, ginger, and curry powder. Heat to a boil. Add pork; cook until tender. Remove from heat. Add lobster. Dissolve cornstarch in cold water. Combine with pork-lobster mixture. Return to heat; thicken slightly. Add bean sprouts. Heat thoroughly. (Add extra water if mixture thickens too much.)

Yield: 1 serving
Exchange: 3 medium-fat meat
Calories: 140

SEAFOOD MEDLEY

1 ounce	chunk tuna	30 grams
1 ounce	small shrimp (cooked)	30 grams
1 teaspoon	lemon juice	5 milliliters
¹/₂	egg (hard cooked & chopped)	¹/₂
1 teaspoon	green onion (sliced)	5 milliliters
1	lettuce leaf	1

Combine all ingredients, except lettuce. Chill thoroughly before serving on lettuce leaf with favorite dressing.

Yield: 1 serving
Exchange: 2¹/₂ medium-fat meat, ¹/₄ vegetable
Calories: 137

BRAN BREAD

3 tablespoons	shortening	45 milliliters
3 tablespoons	brown sugar replacement	45 milliliters
3 tablespoons	molasses	45 milliliters
1 teaspoon	salt	5 milliliters
¹/₂ cup	bran	125 milliliters
³/₄ cup	boiling water	190 milliliters
1 packet	dry yeast	1 packet
¹/₄ cup	warm water	60 milliliters
2¹/₂ cups	flour	625 milliliters
	margarine (melted)	

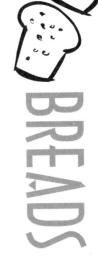

Place shortening, brown sugar replacement, molasses, salt, and bran in large mixing bowl. Add boiling water. Stir to blend. Soften dry yeast in warm water. Allow to rest for 5 minutes. Add yeast to bran mixture. Add flour, 1 cup (250 milliliters) at a time, stirring well between additions, until a soft dough is formed. Knead gently for 10 minutes. Shape into loaf. Place in greased 13 x 9 x 2-inch (33 x 23 x 5-centimeter) loaf pan. Cover; allow to rise for 2 hours. Punch down; allow to rise for 1 hour. Bake at 325°F (165°C) for 50 to 55 minutes. Remove to rack and brush lightly with melted margarine.

> **Yield:** 1 loaf (14 slices)
> **Exchange:** (1 slice) 1 bread
> **Calories:** (1 slice) 68

QUICK ONION BREAD

1 loaf	frozen bread dough	1 loaf
1 package	onion soup mix	1 package

Allow bread to thaw as directed on package. Roll dough out on unfloured board. Sprinkle half of soup mix over surface. Roll up jelly-roll style. Knead to work mix into dough; repeat with remaining soup mix. Form into loaf. Place in greased 9 x 5-inch (23 x 13-centimeter) loaf pan; cover. Allow to rise about 2 hours. Bake at 350°F (175°C) for 30 to 40 minutes, or until done.

> **Yield:** 1 loaf (14 slices)
> **Exchange:** (1 slice) 1 bread
> **Calories:** (1 slice) 80

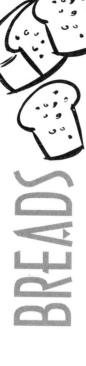

JEWISH BRAID BREAD (CHALLAH)

1 packet	dry yeast	1 packet
³/₄ cup	warm water	190 milliliters
1 teaspoon	salt	5 milliliters
¹/₄ cup	sugar replacement	60 milliliters
2 tablespoons	margarine (melted)	30 milliliters
2	eggs (well beaten)	2
3 cups	flour	750 milliliters
1 teaspoon	skim milk	5 milliliters
	poppy seeds	

Soften yeast in warm water; allow to rest for 5 minutes. Add salt, sugar replacement, and margarine. Measure 1 tablespoon (15 milliliters) of the beaten eggs. Place in cup and reserve. Add remaining eggs and 1 cup (250 milliliters) of the flour to yeast mixture; beat vigorously. Add remaining flour. Turn onto floured board and knead until smooth and elastic. Place in lightly greased bowl; cover. Allow to rise until double in size, about 1¹/₂ hours. Punch down; divide into thirds. Roll into three strips, 18 inches (45 centimeters) long, with the heel of the hand. Braid the 3 strips loosly, tucking under ends. Blend reserved beaten egg with 1 teaspoon (5 milliliters) skim milk, carefully brush over braid. Sprinkle with poppy seeds; cover. Allow to rise until double in size, about 1¹/₂ hours. Bake at 350°F (175°C) for 1 hour, or until done.

Yield: 1 loaf (18 slices)
Exchange: (1 slice) 1 bread
Calories: (1 slice) 70

BAKED SWEET POTATO

¹/₄ cup	sweet potato or yam (mashed)	60 milliliters
dash each	salt, pepper, nutmeg	dash each
1 tablespoon	milk	15 milliliters

Combine all ingredients. Beat until smooth and creamy. Bake at 350°F (175°C) for 20 minutes.

Yield: 1 serving
Exchange: 1 bread
Calories: 75

APRICOT BREAD

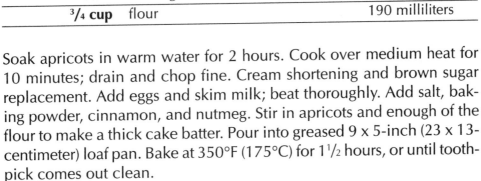

8	dried apricot halves	8
¹/₃ cup	shortening	90 milliliters
¹/₄ cup	brown sugar replacement (packed)	60 milliliters
2	eggs (beaten)	2
1 cup	skim milk	250 milliliters
¹/₂ teaspoon	salt	2 milliliters
1¹/₂ teaspoons	baking powder	7 milliliters
¹/₄ teaspoon	cinnamon	1 milliliter
dash	nutmeg	dash
³/₄ cup	flour	190 milliliters

Soak apricots in warm water for 2 hours. Cook over medium heat for 10 minutes; drain and chop fine. Cream shortening and brown sugar replacement. Add eggs and skim milk; beat thoroughly. Add salt, baking powder, cinnamon, and nutmeg. Stir in apricots and enough of the flour to make a thick cake batter. Pour into greased 9 x 5-inch (23 x 13-centimeter) loaf pan. Bake at 350°F (175°C) for 1¹/₂ hours, or until toothpick comes out clean.

Microwave: Bake on LOW for 20 minutes. Increase heat to HIGH for 5 minutes, or until toothpick comes out clean. Hold 2 minutes. Turn pan a quarter turn every 10 minutes.

> **Yield:** 1 loaf (14 slices)
> **Exchange:** (1 slice) 1 bread, 1 fat
> **Calories:** (1 slice) 75

POPOVERS

1 cup	flour	250 milliliters
¹/₂ teaspoon	salt	2 milliliters
2	eggs	2
1 cup	skim milk	250 milliliters

Sift flour and salt together; set aside. Beat eggs and skim milk; add to flour. Beat until smooth and creamy. Pour into heated greased muffin tins, filling half full or less. Bake at 375°F (190°C) for 50 minutes, or until popovers are golden brown and sound hollow. DO NOT OPEN OVEN FOR FIRST 40 MINUTES!

> **Yield:** 18 popovers
> **Exchange:** (1 popover) ¹/₂ bread, ¹/₈ meat
> **Calories:** (1 popover) 44

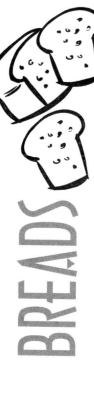

RAISIN BREAD

1 packet	dry yeast	1 packet
¼ cup	warm water	60 milliliters
¾ cup	milk (scalded & cooled)	180 milliliters
2 tablespoons	sugar replacement	30 milliliters
1 teaspoon	salt	5 milliliters
1	egg	1
2 tablespoons	margarine (softened)	30 milliliters
3¾ cups	flour	940 milliliters
1 cup	raisins	250 milliliters

Soften yeast in warm water; allow to rest for 5 minutes. Combine milk, sugar replacement, salt, egg, and margarine; mix thoroughly. Stir in yeast mixture. Add 1 cup (250 milliliters) of the flour. Beat until smooth. Mix in raisins. Blend in remaining flour. Knead for 5 minutes. Cover; allow to rise for 2 hours. Punch down; form into loaf. Place in greased 9 x 5-inch (23 x 13-centimeter) loaf pan; cover. Allow to rise for 1 hour. Bake at 400°F (200°C) for 30 minutes, or until loaf sounds hollow and is golden brown. Remove to rack.

> **Yield:** 1 loaf (14 slices)
> **Exchange:** (1 slice) 1 bread
> **Calories:** (1 slice) 68

SOYA CRISPS

1 cup	soya flour	250 milliliters
1 cup	chicken broth	250 milliliters
1 tablespoon	liquid shortening	15 milliliters
1 teaspoon	salt	5 milliliters

Blend soya flour and broth in saucepan until smooth. Bring gradually to a boil; remove from heat. Blend in liquid shortening and salt. Pour into large flat baking sheet to a depth of no more than ¼ inch (6 millimeters). Bake at 325°F (165°C) for 30 minutes. Cool slightly. Cut into 2¼-inch (6-centimeter) squares. Cut diagonally into triangles.

> **Yield:** 80 chips
> **Exchange:** (10 chips) 1 lean meat
> **Calories:** (10 chips) 50

PIONEER CORNBREAD

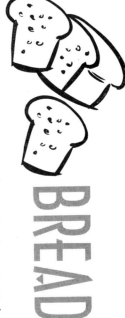

1	egg	1
1 cup	skim milk	250 milliliters
2 tablespoons	lo-cal maple syrup	30 milliliters
2 tablespoons	margarine (melted)	30 milliliters
²/₃ cup	cornmeal	160 milliliters
³/₄ cup	flour	190 milliliters
1 tablespoon	baking powder	30 milliliters
1 teaspoon	salt	5 milliliters

Beat egg until light and lemon colored. Add skim milk, maple syrup, and margarine. Combine cornmeal, flour, baking powder, and salt in large bowl. Stir to blend. Gradually add flour mixture to liquid. Pour into greased 8-inch (20-centimeter) square pan. Bake at 425°F (220°C) for 20 to 25 minutes.

Microwave: Bake on LOW for 10 minutes. Increase heat to HIGH for 5 minutes, or until toothpick comes out clean.

> **Yield:** 9 squares
> **Exchange:** (1 square) 1¹/₂ bread
> **Calories:** (1 square) 82

BAKING POWDER BISCUITS

1 cup	flour	250 milliliters
1 teaspoon	baking powder	5 milliliters
¹/₄ teaspoon	yeast	1 milliliter
¹/₄ teaspoon	salt	1 milliliter
1 tablespoon	liquid shortening	15 milliliters
6 tablespoons	milk	90 milliliters
	vegetable cooking spray	

Combine all ingedients, except vegetable cooking spray; mix just until blended. Turn out on floured board. Roll out to a ¹/₂-inch (1-centimeter) thickness. Cut into circles with floured 2-inch (5-centimeter) cutter. Place on baking sheet coated with vegetable cooking spray; cover. Allow to rest for 10 minutes. Bake at 450°F (230°C) for 12 to 15 minutes, or until lightly browned.

> **Yield:** 10 biscuits
> **Exchange:** (1 biscuit) 1 bread, ¹/₂ fat
> **Calories:** (1 biscuit) 90

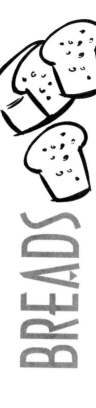

BREADS

YEAST ROLLS

1 packet	dry yeast	1 packet
¼ cup	warm water	60 milliliters
2 tablespoons	sugar replacement	30 milliliters
2 teaspoons	salt	10 milliliters
1 tablespoon	margarine (melted)	15 milliliters
¾ cup	warm water	190 milliliters
3½ cups	flour	875 milliliters
1	egg (well beaten)	1

Soften yeast in the ¼ cup (60 milliliters) warm water. Allow to rest for 5 minutes. Combine sugar replacement, salt, margarine, and the ¾ cup (190 milliliters) warm water; stir to mix. Add 1 cup (250 milliliters) of the flour; beat well. Blend in yeast mixture and the egg. Add remaining flour; mix well. Knead gently until dough is smooth; cover. Allow to rise for 1 hour. Punch down. Allow to rest for 10 minutes. Shape into 36 rolls. Place on greased cookie sheet or in greased muffin tins. Allow to rise until doubled in size, about 1½ to 2 hours. Bake at 400°F (200°C) for 20 to 25 minutes, or until golden brown.

Yield: 36 rolls
Exchange: (1 roll) 1 bread
Calories: (1 roll) 68

FRESH APPLE MUFFINS

2 tablespoons	soft margarine	30 milliliters
2 tablespoons	sugar replacement	30 milliliters
1	egg (beaten)	1
1¼ cups	flour	310 milliliters
¼ teaspoon	salt	1 milliliter
2 teaspoons	baking powder	10 milliliters
6 tablespoons	skim milk	90 milliliters
1 small	apple (peeled & chopped)	1 small

Cream margarine and sugar replacement; add egg. Stir in remaining ingredients. Spoon into greased muffin tins, filling no more than two-thirds full. Bake at 400°F (200°C) for 25 minutes, or until done.

Yield: 12 muffins
Exchange: (1 muffin) 1 bread
Calories: (1 muffin) 72

ORANGE MUFFINS

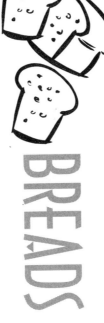

1 cup	orange juice	250 milliliters
1 tablespoon	orange peel (grated)	15 milliliters
1/2 cup	raisins (soaked)	125 milliliters
1/3 cup	sugar replacement	80 milliliters
1 tablespoon	margarine	15 milliliters
1	egg	1
1/4 teaspoon	salt	1 milliliter
1 teaspoon	baking soda	5 milliliters
1 teaspoon	baking powder	5 milliliters
1/2 teaspoon	vanilla extract	2 milliliters
2 cups	flour	500 milliliters

Combine orange juice, orange peel, and raisins. Allow to rest for 1 hour. Cream together the sugar replacement, margarine, and egg. Add salt, baking soda, baking powder, and vanilla extract. Stir in orange juice mixture. Stir in enough of the flour to make a thick cake batter. Spoon into greased muffin tins, filling no more than two-thirds full. Bake at 350°F (175°C) for 20 to 25 minutes, or until done.

Microwave: Spoon into 6-ounce (180-milliliter) custard cups, filling no more that two-thirds full. Cook on LOW for 7 to 8 minutes. Increase heat to HIGH for 2 minutes, or until done.

> **Yield:** 24 muffins
> **Exchange:** (1 muffin) 1 bread
> **Calories:** (1 muffin) 68

POTATO DUMPLINGS

1 small	potato (cooked)	1 small
1	egg (beaten)	1
2 tablespoons	flour	30 milliliters
	salt & pepper to taste	

With a fork, break up and mash the potato. Combine with the remaining ingredients. Beat until light and fluffy. Drop by tablespoonfuls on top of boiling salted water or beef broth. Boil for 5 minutes, or until dumplings rise to surface. Good with Sauerbraten (page 97).

> **Yield:** 3 or 4 dumplings
> **Exchange:** 1 bread, 1 meat
> **Calories:** 140

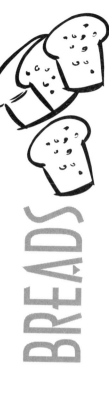

CAKE DOUGHNUTS

1 tablespoon	granulated sugar	15 milliliters
4 tablespoons	sugar replacement	60 milliliters
⅓ cup	buttermilk	80 milliliters
1	egg (well beaten)	1
1 cup	flour	250 milliliters
⅛ teaspoon	baking soda	½ milliliter
1 teaspoon	baking powder	5 milliliters
dash each	nutmeg, cinnamon, vanilla extract, salt	dash each
	oil for deep-fat frying	

Combine sugars, buttermilk, and egg; beat well. Add remaining ingredients, except oil. Beat just until blended. Heat oil to 375°F (190°C). Drop dough from doughnut dropper into hot fat. Fry until golden brown, turning often. Drain.

Yield: 12 doughnuts
Exchange: (1 doughnut) 1 bread, 1 fat
Calories: (1 doughnut) 130

TEA SCONES

1 cup	flour	250 milliliters
1 teaspoon	baking powder	5 milliliters
¼ teaspoon	salt	1 milliliter
1 tablespoon	sugar replacement	15 milliliters
¼ cup	margarine (cold)	60 milliliters
1	egg	1
¼ cup	evaporated (skim) milk	60 milliliters

Sift flour, baking powder, salt, and sugar replacement. Cut in cold margarine as for pie crust. Beat egg and evaporated milk together thoroughly; stir into flour mixture. Knead gently on lightly floured board. Divide dough in half; roll each half into a circle. Cut circles into quarters. Place on lightly greased cookie sheet. Brush tops with milk. Bake at 450°F (230°C) for 15 minutes, or until done.

Yield: 8 scones
Exchange: (1 scone) 1 bread
Calories: (1 scone) 34

SCONE VARIATIONS

Stir one of the following into flour mixture for Tea Scones:

APPLE

8	dried apple halves (chopped)	8

Exchange: (1 scone) 1 bread, ¼ fruit
Calories: (1 scone) 44

APRICOT

8	dried apricot halves (chopped)	8

Exchange: (1 scone) 1 bread, ¼ fruit
Calories: (1 scone) 44

CRANBERRY

¼ cup	cranberries (chopped)	60 milliliters

Exchange: (1 scone) 1 bread
Calories: (1 scone) 34

DATES

8	dates (chopped)	8

Exchange: (1 scone) 1 bread, ½ fruit
Calories: (1 scone) 54

LEMON

1 tablespoon	lemon peel (grated)	15 milliliters

Exchange: (1 scone) 1 bread
Calories: (1 scone) 34

ORANGE

1½ tablespoons	orange peel (grated)	25 milliliters

Exchange: (1 scone) 1 bread
Calories: (1 scone) 34

PEACH

8	dried peach halves (chopped)	8

Exchange: (1 scone) 1 bread, ½ fruit
Calories: (1 scone) 54

RAISIN

4 tablespoons	raisins	60 milliliters

Exchange: (1 scone) 1 bread, ¼ fruit
Calories: (1 scone) 44

BREADS

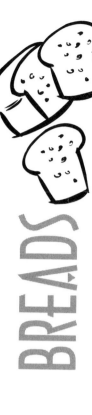

PITA BREAD

1 packet	dry yeast	1 packet
1/2 teaspoon	sugar replacement	2 milliliters
1 teaspoon	salt	5 milliliters
1 tablespoon	liquid shortening	15 milliliters
1 1/2 cups	warm water	375 milliliters
4 cups	flour	1000 milliliters

Dissolve yeast, sugar, salt, and liquid shortening in warm water. Add 3 cups (750 milliliters) of the flour; stir to mix well. (Dough should be fairly stiff; if not, add more flour.) Turn out onto floured surface; knead in remaining flour. (Dough will be very stiff.) Form into 15 1/2-inch (40 - centimeter) tube. Cut into 15 slices. Pat to make circles about 6 inches (15 centimeters) in diameter. Lay on lightly greased baking pans; cover. Allow to rise until almost doubled, about 1 1/2 to 2 hours. Bake 475°F (245°C) for 10 to 12 minutes, or until lightly golden brown, puffed, and hollow. These freeze well.

Yield: 15 pita bread pockets
Exchange: (1 pocket) 1 1/2 bread, 1/2 fat
Calories: (1 pocket) 70

POTATO PANCAKE

1 medium	raw potato (grated)	1 medium
1	egg	1
2 tablespoons	flour	30 milliliters
2 teaspoons	salt	10 milliliters
2 teaspoons	chives	10 milliliters
	vegetable cooking spray	

Place grated potato in ice water. Allow to stand for 30 minutes to an hour. Drain; pat potato dry. Place potato in bowl; add egg, flour, salt, and chives. Stir to blend. Divide mixture into 4 parts and spoon into large skillet coated with vegetable cooking spray. Brown on both sides.

Yield: 4 pancakes
Exchange: (2 pancakes) 1 bread, 1/2 medium-fat meat
Calories: (2 pancakes) 80

MOUNTAIN MAN PANCAKES

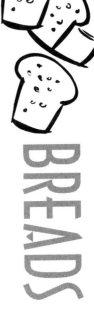

1	egg	1
1¼ cups	buttermilk	310 milliliters
1 tablespoon	molasses	15 milliliters
2 tablespoons	margarine (melted)	30 milliliters
1 cup	flour	250 milliliters
1 teaspoon	salt	5 milliliters
½ teaspoon	baking soda	2 milliliters
2 teaspoons	baking powder	10 milliliters
½ cup	yellow cornmeal	125 milliliters
	vegetable cooking spray	

Beat egg, buttermilk, molasses, and margarine together until well blended. Add remaining ingredients, except vegetable cooking spray. Stir just enough to blend. Cook in skillet coated with vegetable cooking spray.

Yield: 10 panckaes, 4 inches (9 centimeters) in diameter each
Exchange: 1 bread, 1 fat
Calories: 95

POTATO PUFFS

½ cup cooked	potatoes (mashed or whipped)	125 milliliters
1 cup	flour	250 milliliters
1½ teaspoons	baking powder	8 milliliters
½ teaspoon	salt	2 milliliters
1	egg (well beaten)	1
½ cup	milk	125 milliliters
	oil for deep-fat frying	

With a fork, break up and mash enough potatoes to fill a small cup. Combine with remaining ingredients, except oil. Beat well. Heat oil to 375°F (190°C). From tablespoon, drop a walnut-size piece of dough into hot fat. Remove when puff rises to the surface (about 2 to 3 minutes) and is golden brown. Repeat with remaining dough. Drain.

Yield: 24 puffs
Exchange: 1 bread, 1½ fat
Calories: 160

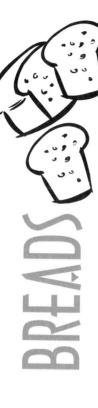

CORNBREAD STUFFING

6 tablespoons	butter	90 milliliters
1 large	onion (chopped)	1 large
1 cup	celery with tops (chopped)	250 milliliters
1 teaspoon	thyme	5 milliliters
1 teaspoon	sage	5 milliliters
1 tablespoon	salt	15 milliliters
1 teaspoon	pepper	5 milliliters
6 cups	cornbread crumbs	1 1/2 liters

Melt butter in medium saucepan. Add onion, celery, thyme, sage, salt, and pepper. Sauté over low heat for 3 to 4 minutes. Remove from heat. Add cornbread crumbs; toss to mix. Add water to moisten to stuffing consistency.

Yield: 6 cups (1 1/2 liters)
Exchange: (1/2 cup/125 milliliters) 1 bread, 1 fat
Calories: (1/2 cup/125 milliliters) 125

HERB-SEASONED STUFFING

1-pound loaf	bread (2 to 3 days old)	500-gram loaf
1/2 cup	butter or margarine	125 milliliters
1 teaspoon	thyme	5 milliliters
1 teaspoon	sage	5 milliliters
1 teaspoon	rosemary	5 milliliters
1 teaspoon	dried lemon rind	5 milliliters

Remove crust from bread; cut bread into cubes. Melt butter or margarine in large skillet. Add seasonings; stir to mix. Add bread cubes. Toss or stir lightly to coat bread cubes. Pour onto baking sheet. Allow to dry by air or dry in very slow oven. These dried bread cubes are good as croutons; add salt and water to moisten when ready to use as stuffing.

Yield: 8 cups (2 liters)
Exchange: (1/2 cup/125 milliliters) 1 bread, 1 fat
Calories: (1/2 cup/125 milliliters) 75

PRUNE-APPLE STUFFING

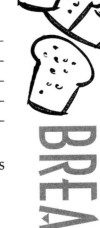

1 cup	prunes (soaked & chopped)	250 milliliters
1¹/₂ cups	apples (chopped)	375 milliliters
¹/₂ cup	raisins	125 milliliters
1 teaspoon	cinnamon	5 milliliters
¹/₂ teaspoon	nutmeg	2 milliliters

Combine fruit and spices; mix thoroughly. Allow to rest for 10 minutes before using.

Yield:	3 cups (750 milliliters)
Exchange:	(¹/₄ cup/60 milliliters) 1 fruit
Calories:	(¹/₄ cup/60 milliliters) 60

BAKED RICE

1 cube	beef bouillon	1 cube
1 cup	hot water	250 millilitres
¹/₄ cup	rice	60 millilitres
1	green onion (chopped)	1
2 tablespoons	celery (chopped)	30 millilitres
3 tablespoons	dry bread crumbs	45 millilitres

Dissolve bouillon in hot water. Add rice, green onion, and celery; cover. Cook for 5 minutes. Add bread crumbs. Pour into small baking dish. Bake at 350°F (175°C) for 25 to 30 minutes, or until top is lightly crusted.

Yield:	1 serving
Exchange:	1¹/₂ bread
Calories:	115

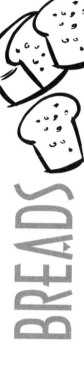

RICE PILAF

¹/₂ cup	rice	125 milliliters
1 teaspoon	butter	5 milliliters
¹/₂ teaspoon	salt	2 milliliters
1 tablespoon	lemon juice	15 milliliters
1 cup	boiling water	250 milliliters

Sauté rice in butter over low heat in large saucepan. Add remaining ingredients. Bring to a boil. Reduce heat; cover. Simmer until water is absorbed. Fluff with fork before serving.

Yield: 1 cup (250 milliliters)
Exchange: 2 bread, 1 fat
Calories: 150

CORN PUDDING

16-ounce can	corn	500-gram can
1	egg (beaten)	1
1 teaspoon	pimiento (chopped)	5 milliliters
1 teaspoon	green pepper	5 milliliters
1 teaspoon	margarine (melted)	5 milliliters
1 teaspoon	sugar replacement	5 milliliters
³/₄ cup	milk	180 milliliters
	salt & pepper to taste	
	vegetable cooking spray	

Combine all ingredients, except vegetable cooking spray. Pour into baking dish coated with vegetable cooking spray. Bake at 325°F (165°C) for 35 to 40 minutes, or until firm.

Yield: 6 servings
Exchange: (1 serving) 1 bread, 1 fat
Calories: (1 serving) 55

ABC's OF VEGETABLES

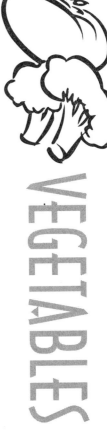

1 cup	asparagus pieces	250 milliliters
1 cup	broccoli florets	250 milliliters
1 cup	carrot slices	250 milliliters
1 cup	spinach (chopped)	250 milliliters
11-ounce can	condensed cream of mushroom soup	300-gram can
2 tablespoons	onions (finely chopped)	30 milliliters
1 teaspoon	thyme	5 milliliters
1/2 cup	water	125 milliliters
	salt & pepper to taste	
	vegetable cooking spray	

Layer asparagus, broccoli, carrots, and spinach in a baking dish coated with vegetable cooking spray. Blend remaining ingredients. Pour over vegetables. Cover. Bake at 350°F (175°C) for 30 to 40 minutes, or until vegetables are tender.

Yield: 8 servings
Exchange: (1 serving) 1 vegetable, 1/2 bread, 1/2 fat
Calories: (1 serving) 42

BAKED EGGPLANT

1 slice	eggplant	1 slice
1 slice	onion	1 slice
1 ounce	sharp Cheddar cheese (shredded)	30 grams
2 tablespoons	condensed tomato soup	30 milliliters
1 teaspoon	dry bread crumbs	5 milliliters
1/4 teaspoon	thyme	1 milliliter
1/4 teaspoon	salt	1 milliliter
dash	pepper	dash

Cook eggplant and onion in small amount of water until tender. Drain; reserve liquid. Place eggplant and onion in small baking dish. Top with cheese. Blend condensed soup, 1 tablespoon (15 milliliters) of the eggplant liquid, bread crumbs, thyme, salt, and pepper. Pour over eggplant; cover. Bake at 350°F (175°C) for 30 minutes.

Microwave: Uncover. Cook on HIGH for 5 minutes. Turn after 2 minutes.

Yield: 1 serving
Exchange: 1 high-fat meat, 1 vegetable
Calories: 161

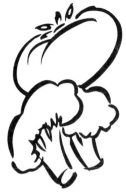

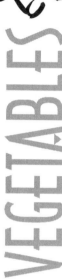

CHEESE TOMATO

1	tomato (thickly sliced)	1
dash each	celery salt, garlic salt, pepper	dash each
1 ounce	American cheese (grated)	30 grams
	vegetable cooking spray	

Place tomato slices on broiler pan coated with vegetable cooking spray. Sprinkle with seasonings. Top with cheese. Broil 5 to 6 inches (15 centimeters) from heat until cheese is melted.

Yield: 1 serving
Exchange: 1 vegetable, 1 high-fat meat
Calories: 140

OKRA AND TOMATOES

2 cups	okra	500 milliliters
¼ cup	vinegar	60 milliliters
2 cups	tomatoes (cut into eighths)	500 milliliters
1 cup	onions (coarsely chopped)	250 milliliters
½ cup	green pepper (coarsely chopped)	125 milliliters
sprig	parsley (chopped)	sprig
1 tablespoon	mint (chopped)	15 milliliters
1 teaspoon	garlic powder	5 milliliters
	salt & pepper to taste	
	vegetable cooking spray	

Soak okra in vinegar for 5 minutes. Drain. Pat okra slightly dry. Combine all ingredients (except vinegar) in baking dish coated with vegetable cooking spray. Cover. Bake at 350°F (175°C) for 45 minutes.

Yield: 5 servings
Exchange: (1 serving) 1 vegetable
Calories: (1 serving) 31

KOHLRABI

2 cups	kohlrabi (cut into strips)	500 milliliters
2 teaspoons	butter (or margarine)	10 milliliters
2 tablespoons	fresh parsley (chopped)	30 milliliters
	salt & pepper to taste	

Cook kohlrabi in boiling salted water until soft; drain. Melt butter or margarine in saucepan. Add parsley; sauté over low heat for 2 minutes. Add kohlrabi. Toss to coat. Add salt and pepper.

> **Yield:** 4 servings
> **Exchange:** (1 serving) 1 vegetable, ½ fat
> **Calories:** (1 serving) 36

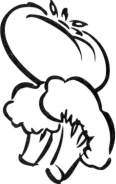

ITALIAN ASPARAGUS

½ pound	asparagus spears (cooked or canned)	250 grams
¼ cup	Tomato Sauce (page 168)	60 milliliters
¼ cup	water	60 milliliters
½ teaspoon	oregano	2 milliliters
¼ teaspoon	garlic powder	1 milliliter
¼ cup	Swiss cheese (grated)	60 milliliters
	salt & pepper to taste	
	vegetable cooking spray	

Lay asparagus spears in shallow baking dish coated with vegetable cooking spray. Blend Tomato Sauce, water, oregano, garlic powder, salt, and pepper. Spread evenly over spears. Top with grated cheese. Bake at 350°F (175°C) for 20 to 25 minutes.

Microwave: Cook on HIGH for 5 to 6 minutes.

> **Yield:** 4 servings
> **Exchange:** (1 serving) ½ vegetable, ½ medium-fat meat
> **Calories:** (1 serving) 58

VEGETABLES

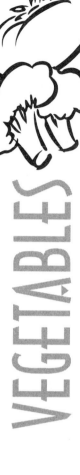

CAULIFLOWER AU GRATIN

2 cups	cauliflower florets	500 milliliters
1 teaspoon	salt	5 milliliters
1 teaspoon	butter	5 milliliters
1 teaspoon	flour	5 milliliters
1 cup	milk (cold)	250 milliliters
1/4 cup	American cheese (diced)	60 milliliters
	salt & pepper to taste	
	vegetable cooking spray	

Place cauliflower florets in large kettle. Fill with enough water to cover. Add salt. Bring to a boil; cook 5 minutes. Drain; rinse with cold water. Melt butter or margarine in saucepan. Blend flour with cold milk. Add to melted butter. Cook over low heat, stirring constantly, until slightly thickened. Add cheese; cook until cheese is completly blended. Place cauliflower in baking dish coated with vegetable cooking spray; add salt and pepper. Cover with cheese topping. Bake at 350°F (175°C) for 20 minutes.

      Yield: 4 servings
Exchange: (1 serving) 1 vegetable, 1/2 medium-fat meat
  Calories: (1 serving) 119

BRUSSELS SPROUTS AND MUSHROOMS AU GRATIN

1 tablespoon	butter	15 milliliters
2 cups	brussels sprouts	500 milliliters
1 cup	mushroom pieces	250 milliliters
2 ounces	Swiss cheese (grated)	60 grams
	salt & pepper to taste	

Melt butter in skillet. Lightly sauté brussels sprouts and mushrooms. Add salt and pepper. Remove from heat and pour into baking dish. Cover with cheese. Bake at 350°F (175°C) for 20 to 25 minutes.

Microwave: Cook on MEDIUM for 10 minutes. Turn once.

      Yield: 4 servings
Exchange: (1 serving) 1 high-fat meat, 1/2 vegetable
  Calories: (1 serving) 65

BAKED VEGETABLE MEDLEY

1 cup	2-inch (5-centimeter) cubes eggplant	250 milliliters
1 cup	2-inch (5-centimeter) slices okra	250 milliliters
1 cup	bean sprouts	250 milliliters
¹/₂ cup	small mushrooms	125 milliliters
1	onion (cut into eighths)	1
11-ounce can	condensed cream of celery soup	300-gram can
¹/₄ cup	water	60 milliliters
1 slice	bread (finely crumbled)	1 slice
	salt & pepper to taste	
	vegetable cooking spray	

Combine all vegetables in baking dish coated with vegetable cooking spray. Blend condensed soup and water; add salt and pepper. Pour over vegetables. Top with bread crumbs. Cook at 325°F (165°C) for 25 to 30 minutes, or until hot, and crumbs are golden brown.

Yield: 8 servings
Exchange: (1 serving) 1 vegetable, ¹/₂ bread
Calories: (1 serving) 49

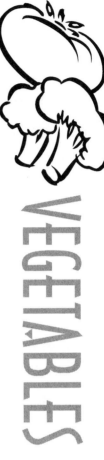

SHREDDED CABBAGE

1 head	cabbage (coarsely shredded)	1 head
2 teaspoons	butter	10 milliliters
¹/₂ teaspoon	nutmeg	2 milliliters
	salt & pepper to taste	

Cook cabbage in a small amount of boiling salted water until tender; drain. Press out excess moisture or pat dry. Melt butter in skillet. Add nutmeg; stir to blend. Add cabbage; toss to coat. Add salt and pepper.

Yield: 4 servings
Exchange: (1 serving) ¹/₂ vegetable, ¹/₂ fat
Calories: (1 serving) 32

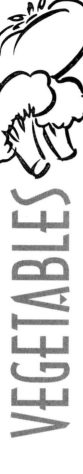

IRISH VEGETABLES

1	bay leaf	1
1 cup	water	250 milliliters
2 tablespoons	wine vinegar	30 milliliters
1/2 cup	corn	125 milliliters
1/2 cup	celery (sliced)	125 milliliters
1/2 cup	broccoli florets	125 milliliters
1/2 cup	carrot (sliced)	125 milliliters
1/2 cup	cauliflowerets	125 milliliters
1/4 cup	pimiento (chopped)	60 milliliters
	salt & pepper to taste	

Combine bay leaf, water, and wine vinegar in medium saucepan. Bring to a boil; add vegetables. Simmer until vegetables are tender. Drain; remove bay leaf. Add salt and pepper.

Yield: 5 servings
Exchange: (1 serving) 1 bread
Calories: (1 serving) 51

SPICED BEAN SPROUTS

2 cups	bean sprouts	500 milliliters
1/2 teaspoon	caraway seeds	2 milliliters
1/2 teaspoon	basil	2 milliliters
2 teaspoons	butter	10 milliliters
	salt & pepper to taste	

Combine bean sprouts, caraway seeds, and basil in saucepan with small amount of water. Cook until hot and tender; drain. Place in serving dish; top with butter, salt and pepper. Toss to coat.

Yield: 4 servings
Exchange: (1 serving) 1/4 vegetable, 1/2 fat
Calories: (1 serving) 25

GERMAN GREEN BEANS

2 cups	green beans	500 milliliters
1 slice	bacon	1 slice
1/4 cup	onion (chopped)	60 milliliters
1 teaspoon	flour	5 milliliters
1/4 cup	vinegar	60 milliliters
1/2 cup	water	125 milliliters
2 tablespoons	sugar replacement	30 milliliters

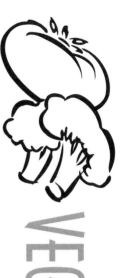

Cook green beans in boiling salted water until tender; drain. Cut bacon into 1/2-inch (12-millimeter) pieces. Place in skillet; add onion. Sauté until bacon is crisp and onion is tender; drain. Blend flour, vinegar, water, and sugar replacement in screwtop jar. Pour over bacon and onion. Cook over low heat to thicken slightly. Add green beans.

Yield: 4 servings
Exchange: (1 serving) 1/2 vegetable, 1/4 bread, 1/2 fat
Calories: (1 serving) 52

PIZZA BEANS

2 cups	green beans	500 milliliters
1 tablespoon	lemon juice	15 milliliters
1/4 teaspoon	oregano	1 milliliter
1 teaspoon	pimiento (chopped)	5 milliliters
dash each	garlic powder, salt	dash each

Cook green beans in boiling salted water until tender; drain. Combine lemon juice, oregano, pimiento, garlic powder, and salt. Pour over beans; toss.

Yield: 5 servings
Exchange: (1 serving) 1 vegetable
Calories: (1 serving) 32

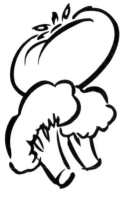

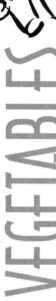

WHIPPED SUMMER SQUASH

3 cups	summer squash	750 milliliters
¼ cup	evaporated milk	60 milliliters
2 teaspoons	butter	10 milliliters
	salt & pepper to taste	

Peel and cut squash into small pieces. Place in saucepan with small amount of water. Bring to a boil; reduce heat and simmer until squash is crisp-tender. Drain. Beat squash with rotary beater; add evaporated milk and butter. Beat until light and fluffy. Add salt and pepper.

Yield: 4 servings
Exchange: (1 serving) 1 vegetable, 1 fat
Calories: (1 serving) 68

SPICED BEETS

½ cup	wine vinegar	125 milliliters
¼ cup	water	60 milliliters
1	bay leaf	1
1	whole clove	1
1 teaspoon	black pepper	5 milliliters
3 tablespoons	sugar replacement	45 milliliters
2 cups	beets (sliced)	500 milliliters

Combine all ingredients except beets. Bring to a boil. Add beets; simmer for 10 minutes, or until tender.

Microwave: Combine all ingredients, except beets. Cook on HIGH for 2 minutes. Add beets. Cook on MEDIUM for 2 minutes.

Yield: 4 servings
Exchange: (1 serving) 1 bread
Calories: (1 serving) 36

INDIAN SQUASH

2 cups	acorn squash (cubed)	500 milliliters
2 teaspoons	margarine	10 milliliters
1 teaspoon	orange rind	5 milliliters
1/4 cup	orange juice	60 milliliters
2 tablespoons	sugar replacement	30 milliliters

Cook squash in small amount of boiling water until crisp-tender; drain. Melt margarine in saucepan. Add orange rind, juice, and sugar replacement. Cook over low heat until sugar is dissolved. Add squash; cover. Continue cooking until squash is tender.

Yield: 4 servings
Exchange: (1 serving) 1 bread, 1/2 fat
Calories: (1 serving) 60

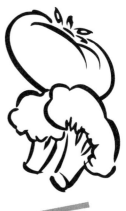

BEANS ORIENTALE

1 1/2 cups	French-cut green beans (cooked)	375 milliliters
2 tablespoons	almonds (blanched & slivered)	30 milliliters
1/2 cup	mushroom pieces	125 milliliters
2 teaspoons	butter	10 milliliters
	salt & pepper to taste	

Heat green beans; drain. Sauté almonds and mushrooms in butter. Add green beans. Add salt and pepper.

Microwave: Melt butter in bowl. Add almonds and mushrooms. Cover. Cook on HIGH for 30 seconds. Add green beans. Cook on MEDIUM for 2 to 3 minutes.

Yield: 4 servings
Exchange: (1 serving) 1/2 vegetable, 1/2 fat
Calories: (1 serving) 45

VEGETABLES

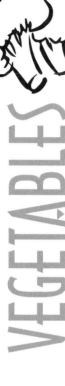

VEGETABLE CASSEROLE

1 cup	peas	250 milliliters
1 cup	green beans	250 milliliters
1 cup	carrots (sliced)	250 milliliters
1 cup	mushrooms	250 milliliters
1	egg	1
1 teaspoon	margarine (melted)	5 milliliters
1/2 cup	milk	125 milliliters
	salt & pepper to taste	
	vegetable cooking spray	

Cook vegetables in small amount of boiling salted water until crisp-tender; drain. Chop vegetables fine. Whip egg until lemon colored; add margarine and milk. Blend well. Add chopped vegetables, salt and pepper. Pour into baking dish coated with vegetable cooking spray. Cover. Bake at 350°F (175°C) for 45 minutes, or until set.

Yield:	8 servings
Exchange:	(1 serving) 1 vegetable
Calories:	(1 serving) 36

PEA POD—CARROT SAUTÉ

1 cup	pea pods	250 milliliters
1 cup	carrots (sliced)	250 milliliters
1 teaspoon	salt	5 milliliters
2 teaspoons	margarine	10 milliliters
1 tablespoon	Worcestershire sauce	15 milliliters

Combine pea pods and carrots in saucepan. Cover with water; add salt. Cook until tender; drain. Melt margarine in saucepan. Add Worcestershire sauce; stir to blend. Add pea pods and carrots. Toss to coat.

Yield:	4 servings
Exchange:	(1 serving) 1/2 bread, 1/2 fat
Calories:	(1 serving) 50

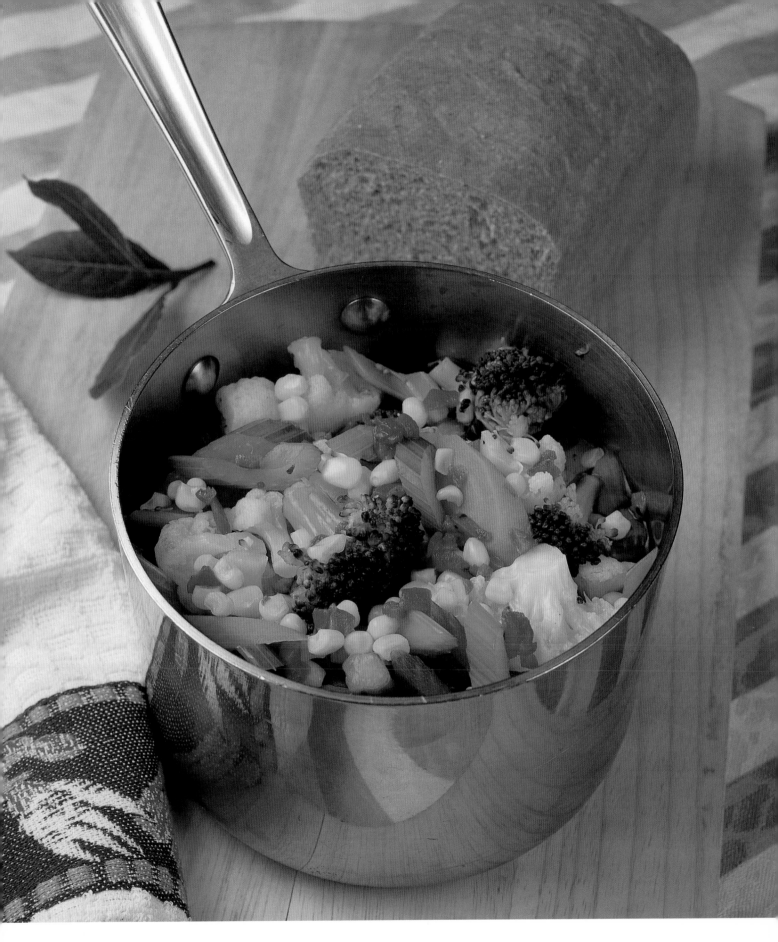

Irish Vegetables

• • •

see page 156

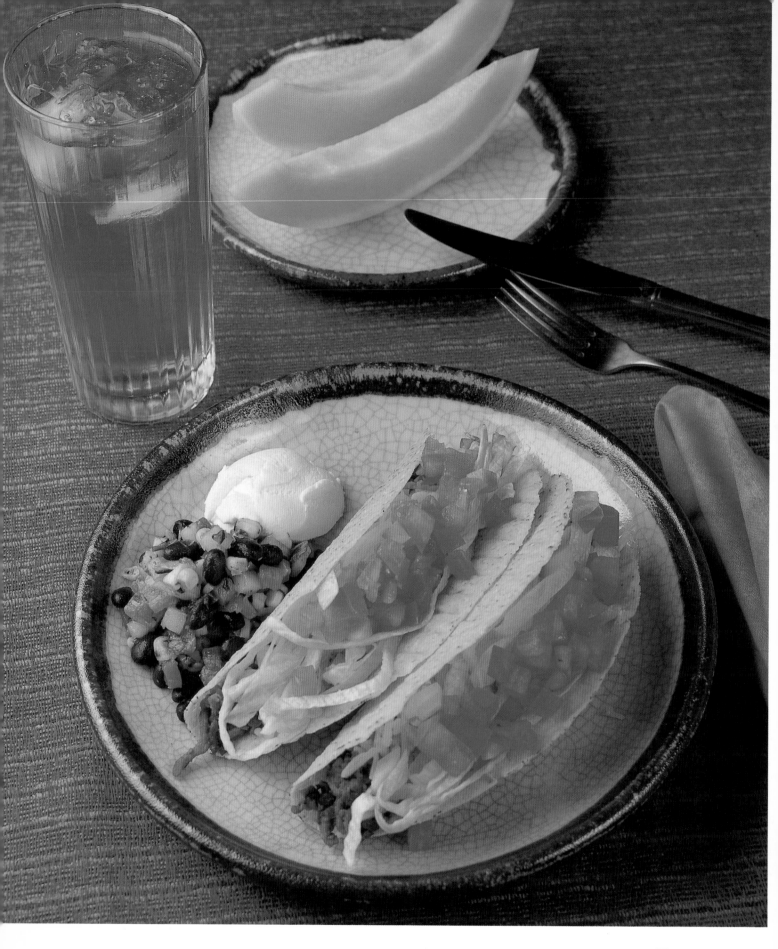

Tacos

• • •

see page 173

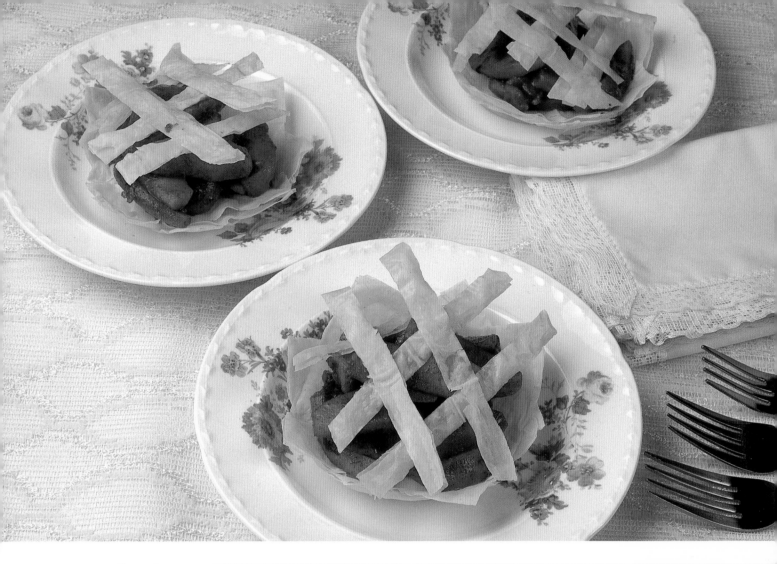

Apple Pie Filling for Pie or Tarts
● ● ●
see page 185

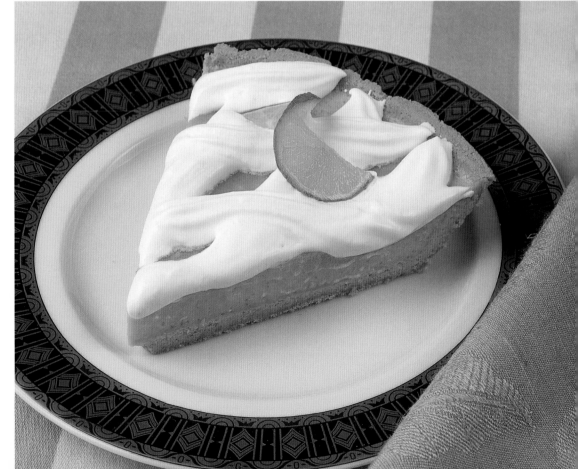

Marion's Lime Pie Filling
● ● ●
see page 190

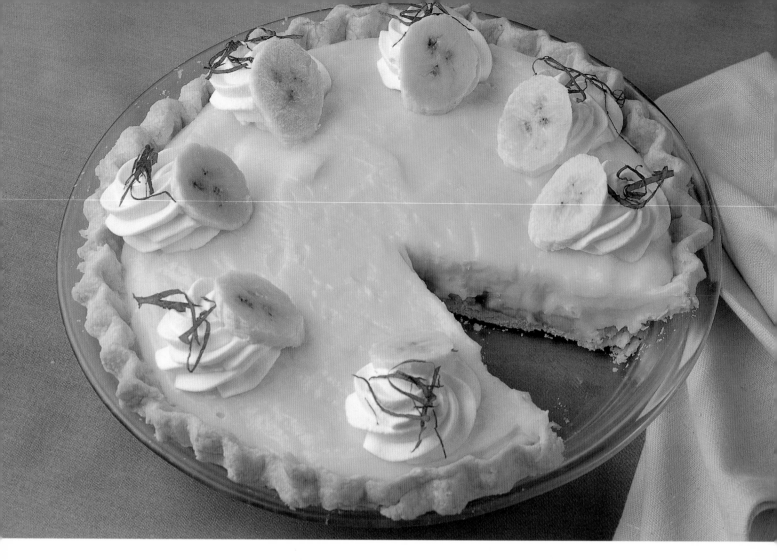

Quick Banana Cream Pie Filling

• • •

see page 191

Rich Chocolate Cake

• • •

see page 203

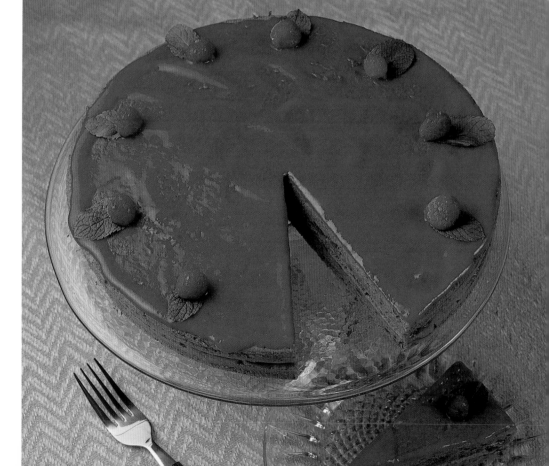

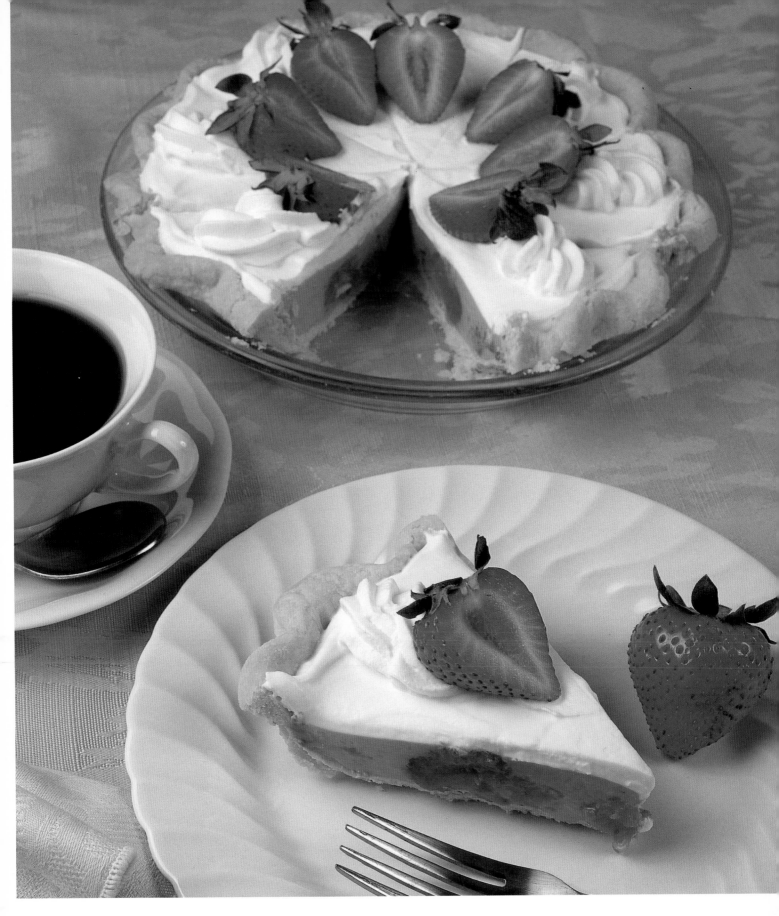

**Luscious Strawberry
Pie Filling**

• • •

see page 193

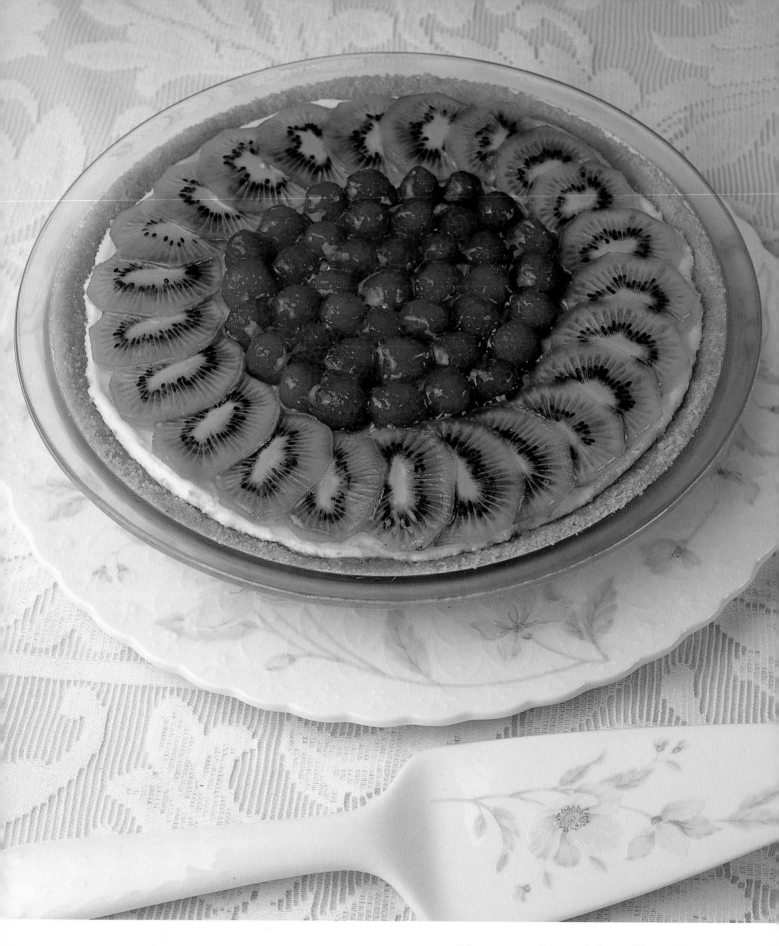

Cheesecake with Jelly Glaze

● ● ●

see page 210

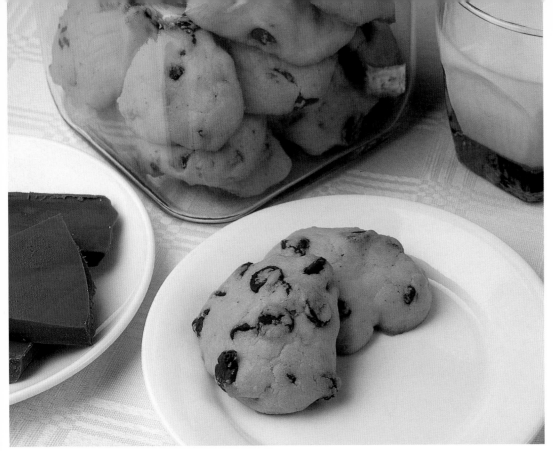

Chocolate Chip Cookies

• • •

see page 216

Pumpkin Bars

• • •

see page 218

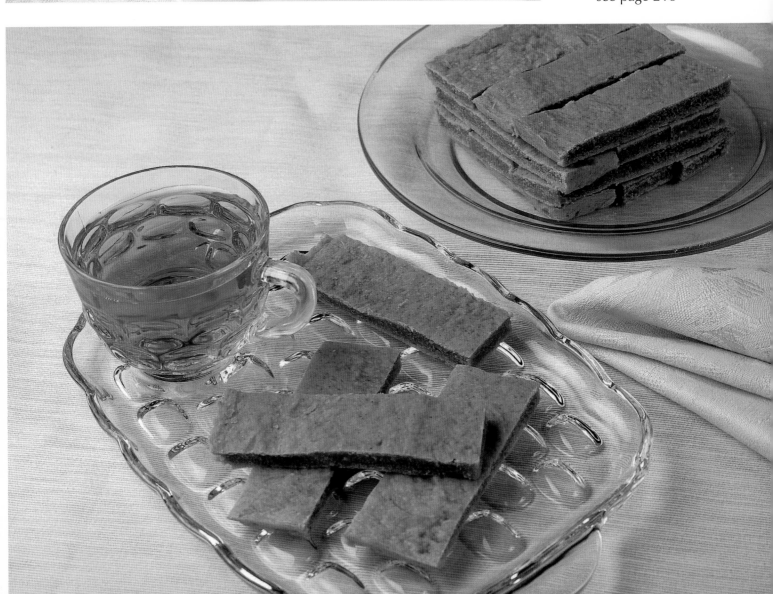

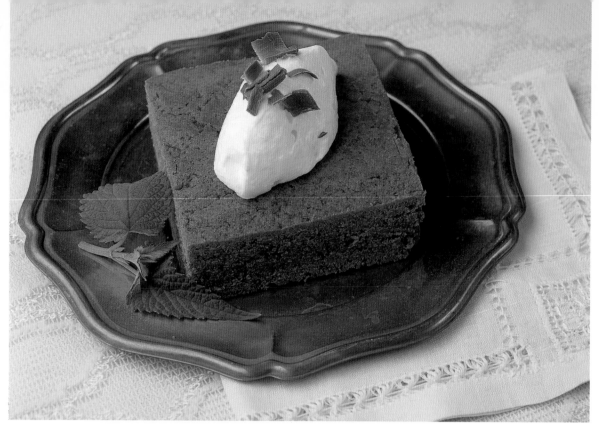

Brownies
• • •
see page 220

Crepes
• • •
see page 231

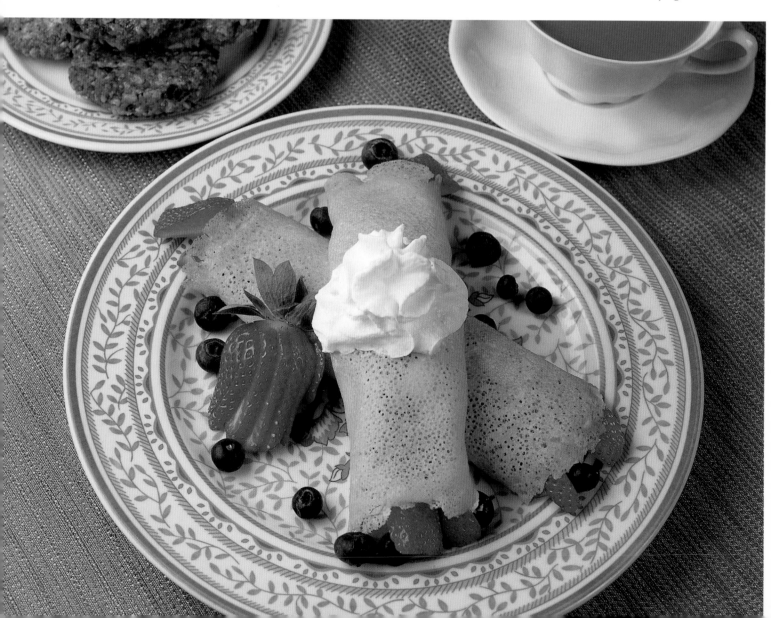

CIRCUS CARROTS

2 cups	carrots (finger- or julienne-cut)	500 milliliters
2 teaspoons	butter	10 milliliters
2 tablespoons	lemon juice	30 milliliters
2 teaspoons	parsley flakes	10 milliliters

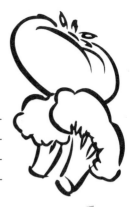

Cook carrots in boiling salted water until tender; keep warm. Melt butter; add lemon juice and parsley flakes. Add warm carrots; toss to coat.

Microwave: Cook carrots in small amount of water on HIGH for 2 minutes. Drain. Add remaining ingredients. Cover. Cook on HIGH for 2 minutes. Toss to mix.

> **Yield:** 4 servings
> **Exchange:** (1 serving) 1 bread, ¼ fat
> **Calories:** (1 serving) 59

CANDIED CARROT SQUARES

4	carrots	4
1 teaspoon	salt	5 milliliters
2 tablespoons	brown sugar replacement	30 milliliters
2 teaspoons	butter	10 milliliters
½ cup	lo-cal cream (or any white) soda	125 milliliters

Cut carrots into lengths to make squares. Place carrots in saucepan and cover with water; add salt. Cook until crisp-tender; drain. Place in baking dish. Sprinkle carrots with brown sugar replacement; dot with butter; add white soda. Bake at 350°F (175°C) for 30 minutes. Turn carrots gently two or three times during baking.

> **Yield:** 4 servings
> **Exchange:** (1 serving) 1 bread, ½ fat
> **Calories:** (1 serving) 47

VEGETABLES

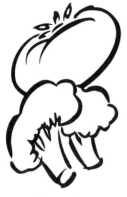

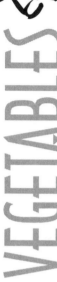

VEGETABLES

SPINACH WITH ONION

2 pounds	fresh spinach	1 kilogram
2 teaspoons	margarine	10 milliliters
1/2 cup	onion (sliced)	125 milliliters
dash each	nutmeg, thyme, salt, pepper	dash each

Rinse spinach thoroughly; place in top of double boiler and heat until wilted. Drain and chop coarsely. Melt margarine in skillet; add onion. Sauté over high heat until onion is brown on the edges. Add seasonings. Stir to blend. Add spinach and toss to blend.

Yield: 4 servings
Exchange: (1 serving) 1/2 vegetable, 1/2 fat
Calories: (1 serving) 37

ZUCCHINI FLORENTINE

4 small	zucchini	4 small
2 teaspoons	margarine	10 milliliters
1 cup	fresh spinach (chopped)	250 milliliters
1 cup	skim milk	250 milliliters
3	eggs (slightly beaten)	3
1 teaspoon	salt	5 milliliters
1/4 teaspoon	pepper	1 milliliter
1/4 teaspoon	thyme	1 milliliter
1/4 teaspoon	paprika	1 milliliter

Cut zucchini into thin slices. Melt margarine in baking dish; add zucchini. Bake at 400°F (200°C) for 15 minutes. Add spinach. Blend skim milk, eggs, salt, pepper, and thyme. Pour over vegetables. Sprinkle with paprika. Bake at 350°F (175°C) for 40 minutes, or until set.

Yield: 6 servings
Exchange: (1 serving) 1 vegetable, 1/2 high-fat meat
Calories: (1 serving) 82

ZUCCHINI WEDGES

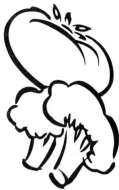

4 small	zucchini	4 small
2 teaspoons	margarine	10 milliliters
2 teaspoons	onion (grated)	10 milliliters
1 cube	beef bouillon	1 cube
2 tablespoons	boiling water	30 milliliters

Cut zucchini in half and lengthwise. Melt margarine in skillet. Add onion and bouillon cube. Press bouillon cube against bottom of skillet to crush. Stir to blend. Place zucchini, cut side down, in skillet. Sauté until golden brown; turn. Add boiling water; cover. Cook over low heat for 10 minutes, or until tender.

Yield: 4 servings
Exchange: (1 serving) $\frac{1}{2}$ vegetable, $\frac{1}{2}$ fat
Calories: (1 serving) 37

VEGETABLES

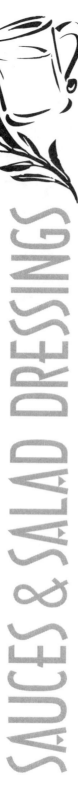

HOLLANDAISE SAUCE

1	egg yolk	1
1 tablespoon	evaporated milk (regular or skim)	15 milliliters
1/8 teaspoon	salt	1/2 milliliter
dash	cayenne pepper	dash
1 tablespoon	lemon juice	15 milliliters
1 tablespoon	margarine	15 milliliters

In the top of a double boiler, heat egg yolk, evaporated milk, salt, and cayenne pepper until thick. Place over hot water. Beat lemon juice into egg mixture until thick and creamy. Remove double boiler from heat. Add margarine, 1 teaspoon (5 milliliters) at a time. Beat until margarine is melted and blended in.

Yield: 1/2 cup (125 milliliters)
Exchange: 1/2 high-fat meat, 3 fat
Calories: 213

WHITE SAUCE

2 tablespoons	margarine	30 milliliters
1 1/2 tablespoons	flour	22 1/2 milliliters
1/4 teaspoon	salt	1 milliliter
1 teaspoon	Worcestershire sauce	5 milliliters
1 cup	skim milk	250 milliliters

Melt margarine. Add flour, salt, and Worcestershire sauce. Blend thoroughly. Add skim milk. Cook until slightly thickened.

Yield: 1 cup (250 milliliters)
Exchange: (1/2 cup/125 milliliters) 1 bread; 1/2 high-fat meat
Calories: (1/2 cup/125 milliliters) 190

ORANGE SAUCE

1/2 teaspoon	cornstarch	2 milliliters
2 tablespoons	cold water	30 milliliters
1/2 cup	orange juice concentrate	125 milliliters
2 teaspoons	unsweetened orange drink mix	10 milliliters

Dissolve cornstarch in cold water. Add orange juice concentrate and drink mix. Cook over low heat until slightly thickened. Use as glaze on poultry or pork.

Yield: 1/2 cup (125 milliliters)
Exchange: 1 fruit
Calories: 52

TERIYAKI MARINADE

1/3 cup	soy sauce	80 milliliters
2 tablespoons	wine vinegar	30 milliliters
2 tablespoons	sugar replacement	30 milliliters
2 teaspoons	salt	10 milliliters
1 teaspoon	ginger (powdered)	5 milliliters
1/2 teaspoon	garlic powder	2 milliliters

Blend well. No calories.

CREOLE SAUCE

28-ounce can	tomatoes	800-gram can
1 medium	onion (chopped)	1 medium
1	green pepper	1
1 teaspoon	paprika	5 milliliters
1/4 teaspoon	marjoram	1 milliliter
	salt & pepper to taste	

Combine all ingredients and cook over low heat for 25 minutes.

Yield: 2 cups (500 milliliters)
Exchange: 1 vegetable
Calories: 25

SAUCES & SALAD DRESSINGS

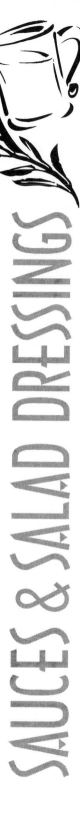

CHILI SAUCE

28-ounce can	tomatoes	800-gram can
1 medium	apple	1 medium
1 medium	onion	1 medium
1 small	green pepper	1 small
1 cup	wine vinegar	250 milliliters
¹/₂ cup	sugar replacement	125 milliliters
1 tablespoon	salt	15 milliliters
¹/₂ teaspoon	ground clove	2 milliliters
¹/₂ teaspoon	cinnamon	2 milliliters
¹/₂ teaspoon	nutmeg	2 milliliters

Mash tomatoes; pour into kettle. Grind together apple, onion, green pepper, and vinegar. Add to kettle; cook until thick. Remove from heat. Add sugar replacement and seasonings. Return to heat; cook 5 minutes, stirring constantly.

Yield: 2 cups (500 milliliters)
Exchange: (¹/₂ cup/125 milliliters) 1 fruit
Calories: (¹/₂ cup/125 milliliters) 45

TANGY BARBECUE SAUCE

1 cup	Chili Sauce (above)	250 milliliters
2 tablespoons	lemon juice	30 milliliters
1 tablespoon	Worcestershire sauce	15 milliliters
1 teaspoon	horseradish	5 milliliters
1 teaspoon	Dijon mustard	5 milliliters
1 tablespoon	brown sugar replacement	15 milliliters
dash each	hot pepper sauce, soy sauce, salt, pepper	dash each

Combine all ingredients; stir to blend well.

Yield: 1 cup (250 milliliters)
Exchange: 2 fruit
Calories: 90

QUICK TOMATO SAUCE

1 cup	catsup	250 milliliters
¹/₂ cup	chili sauce	125 milliliters
2 tablespoons	Worcestershire sauce	30 milliliters
1 tablespoon	water	15 milliliters
1 teaspoon	Dijon-style mustard	5 milliliters
1 teaspoon	yellow mustard	5 milliliters
1 teaspoon	cider vinegar	5 milliliters
¹/₂ teaspoon	black pepper	2 milliliters
¹/₈ teaspoon	mace	¹/₂ milliliter

Combine all ingredients in a bowl; stir to completely blend. Store in airtight container. Heat before using.

Yield:	1¹/₂ cups (375 milliliters) or 22 servings
Exchange:	(1 serving) 1 vegetable
Calories:	(1 serving) 20
Carbohydrates:	(1 serving) 5 grams

ITALIAN TOMATO SAUCE

6	tomatoes (peeled & cubed)	6
¹/₄ cup	green pepper (chopped)	60 milliliters
¹/₄ cup	onion (chopped)	60 milliliters
2 tablespoons	parsley (chopped)	30 milliliters
1 tablespoon	lemon juice	15 milliliters
dash each	oregano, marjoram, thyme, crushed bay leaf, horseradish	dash each
	salt & pepper to taste	

Combine all ingredients in blender. Whip until smooth. Add enough water to make 2 cups (500 milliliters).

Yield:	2 cups (500 milliliters)
Exchange:	2 vegetable
Calories:	10

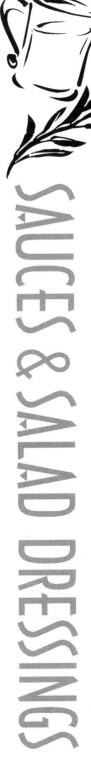

SAUCES & SALAD DRESSINGS

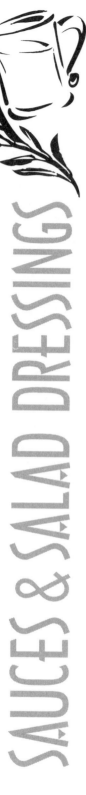

TOMATO SAUCE

firm red tomatoes (or canned
tomatoes without seasonings)

Quarter the tomatoes. Place in large kettle. Push down with hands or back of spoon to render some juice. Bake at 325°F (165°C) until soft pulp remains. Spoon into blender. Blend until smooth. Seal in sterilized jars or freeze.

SWEET YOGURT DRESSING

1 cup	lo-cal yogurt	250 milliliters
¹/₂ teaspoon	mace	2 milliliters
2 teaspoons	sugar replacement	10 milliliters
dash	salt	dash
¹/₂ cup	lo-cal whipped topping (prepared)	125 milliliters

Drain yogurt; beat until smooth and fluffy. Add mace, sugar replacement, and salt. Beat until blended. Fold in prepared whipped topping. Place in refrigerator until ready to serve. Good on fruit or gelatin salads.

Yield: 1 cup (250 milliliters)
Exchange: 1 milk
Calories: 100

HERB YOGURT DRESSING

1 cup	lo-cal yogurt	250 milliliters
2 tablespoons	vinegar	30 milliliters
1 teaspoon	onion (grated)	5 milliliters
1 teaspoon	celery seeds	5 milliliters
1 teaspoon	dry mustard	5 milliliters
1 teaspoon	salt	5 milliliters
¹/₂ teaspoon	thyme	2 milliliters
	salt & pepper to taste	

Beat yogurt until smooth. Add remaining ingredients; blend well. Cover. Allow to rest at least 1 hour before serving.

Yield: 1 cup (250 milliliters)
Exchange: 1 milk
Calories: 86

SALAD DRESSING

1¹/₂ cups	cold water	375 milliliters
¹/₄ cup	vinegar	60 milliliters
1¹/₂ teaspoons	salt	7 milliliters
1 teaspoon	yellow mustard	5 milliliters
2 tablespoons	flour	30 milliliters
1	egg (well beaten)	1
¹/₄ cup	sugar replacement	60 milliliters
2 teaspoons	margarine	10 milliliters

Combine cold water, vinegar, salt, mustard, flour, and egg in top of double boiler. Stir to blend. Cook until thick. Remove from heat. Add sugar replacement and margarine. Stir to blend.

Yield: 1 cup (250 milliliters)
Exchange: (2 tablespoons/30 milliliters) ¹/₂ vegetable, ¹/₂ fat
Calories: (2 tablespoons/30 milliliters) 31

BAY SALAD DRESSING

3 tablespoons	liquid shortening	45 milliliters
¹/₂ cup	onion (finely chopped)	125 milliliters
2 tablespoons	fresh parsley (finely chopped)	30 milliliters
2 tablespoons	celery with leaves (finely chopped)	30 milliliters
1	bay leaf	1
dash each	thyme, mace, rosemary	dash each
2 tablespoons	white wine	30 milliliters
1 cup	yogurt	250 milliliters
2 tablespoons	skim milk	30 milliliters
	salt & pepper to taste	

Heat liquid shortening in small skillet. Add onion, parsley, celery and seasonings. Cook over very low heat, stirring constantly, for 15 minutes. DO NOT ALLOW VEGETABLES TO BURN. Set aside to cool. Add wine; stir to mix. Allow to rest 30 minutes. Strain; reserving liquid. Beat yogurt with skim milk. Continue beating, adding wine liquid. Add salt and pepper. Blend.

Yield: 1¹/₂ cup (375 milliliters)
Exchange: (¹/₄ cup/60 milliliters) ¹/₂ vegetable, ¹/₂ fat
Calories: (¹/₄ cup/60 milliliters) 44

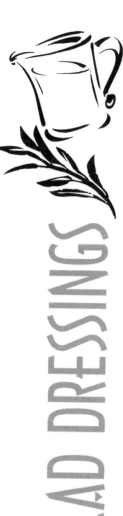

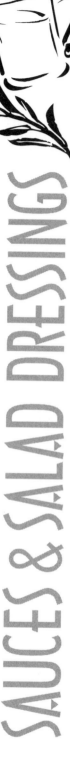

SAUCES & SALAD DRESSINGS

VARIATIONS FOR ITALIAN DRESSING

To ¹/₂ cup (125 milliliters) lo-cal Italian dressing, add:

ANCHOVY

1 ounce	anchovy fillets (mashed)	30 grams
Exchange:	1 meat	

BACON

1 tablespoon	Bacos (ground) (allow to mellow several hours)	15 milliliters
Exchange:	¹/₂ fat	

PARMESAN

1 tablespoon	Parmesan cheese (allow to mellow several hours)	15 milliliters
Exchange:	¹/₈ meat	

TOMATO

1 tablespoon	Tomato puree	15 milliliters

WINE

1 tablespoon	dry white or red wine	15 milliliters
Calories:	(¹/₂ cup/125 milliliters) 24	

VARIATIONS FOR FRENCH DRESSING

To ¹/₂ cup (125 milliliters) lo-cal French dressing, add:

AVOCADO

2 tablespoons	avocado (mashed)	30 milliliters
Exchange:	1 fat	

CHEESE

2 tablespoons	Bleu or Roquefort cheese (mashed)	30 milliliters
Exchange:	¹/₄ meat	

EGG

1 hard-cooked   egg yolk (crumbled)   1 hard-cooked
(combine with dash of hot pepper sauce)

Exchange: 1 meat

LEMON

1 tablespoon   lemon juice   15 milliliters

SOY SAUCE

1 tablespoon   soy sauce   15 milliliters

Calories: (¹/₂ cup/125 milliliters) 100

VARIATIONS
FOR BLEU CHEESE DRESSING

To ¹/₂ cup (125 milliliters) lo-cal Bleu cheese dressing, add:

ANCHOVY

1 ounce   anchovy fillets (mashed)   30 grams

Exchange: 1 meat

BACON

1 tablespoon   Bacos (ground)   15 milliliters
(allow to mellow several hours)

Exchange: ¹/₂ fat

CHIVE

2 tablespoons   chives (chopped)   30 milliliters
(allow to mellow several hours)

HERB

1 teaspoon each   ground parsley, chives, marjoram   5 milliliters

Calories: (¹/₂ cup/125 milliliters) 56

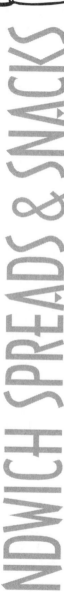

BEEF TONGUE SPREAD

6 ounces	cooked beef tongue (chopped)	180 grams
2 tablespoons	Chili Sauce (page 166)	30 milliliters
1 tablespoon	onion (finely chopped)	15 milliliters

Combine all ingredients; blend well.

Yield: 1 cup (250 milliliters)
Exchange: (¼ cup/60 milliliters) 1 medium-fat meat
Calories: (¼ cup/60 milliliters) 76

SWEET SPREAD

½ cup	margarine	125 milliliters
1 teaspoon	cinnamon	5 milliliters
1 teaspoon	orange rind (grated)	5 milliliters
½ teaspoon	nutmeg	2 milliliters
2 tablespoons	sugar replacement	30 milliliters

Have margarine at room temperature. Beat until light and fluffy. Add remaining ingredients. Beat until blended.

Yield: 24 servings
Exchange: (1 teaspoon/5 milliliters) 1 fat
Calories: (1 teaspoon/5 milliliters) 45

WALDORF SANDWICH SPREAD

¼ cup	celery (finely chopped)	60 milliliters
1 small	apple (finely chopped)	1 small
1 tablespoon	raisins (finely chopped)	15 milliliters
6 halves	walnuts (finely chopped)	6 halves
2 tablespoons	Salad Dressing (page 169)	30 milliliters
	salt to taste	

Combine all ingredients; blend well.

Yield: ½ cup (125 milliliters)
Exchange: (¼ cup/60 milliliters) 1 fruit, 1 fat
Calories: (¼ cup/60 milliliters) 96

TACOS

3 ounces	lean ground beef	90 grams
1 tablespoon	taco sauce	15 milliliters
3	6-inch (15 centimeter) taco shells	3
1 1/2 ounces	Cheddar cheese (grated)	45 grams
1 1/2 tablespoons	onion (chopped)	22 1/2 milliliters
1 medium	tomato (chopped)	1 medium
1 cup	lettuce (shredded)	250 milliliters
	salt & pepper to taste	

Brown beef over low heat. Add salt and pepper. Drain. Add taco sauce; mix well. Divide beef mixture evenly among warm crisp shells. Top with cheese, onion, tomato, and lettuce.

Yield: 1 serving
Exchange: 1 bread, 4 1/2 meat, 1 vegetable
Calories: (1 taco) 145

TUNA SPREAD

6 1/2-ounce can	tuna (in water)	200-milliliter can
2 tablespoons	onion (finely choppd)	30 milliliters
2 tablespoons	celery (finely choppd)	30 milliliters
1 tablespoon	carrot (finely choppd)	15 milliliters
1/4 cup	lo-cal bleu cheese dressing	60 milliliters
	salt & pepper to taste	

Drain tuna; chop fine. Add remaining ingredients and mix well.

Yield: 1 cup (250 milliliters)
Exchange: (1/4 cup/60 milliliters) 1 lean meat
Calories: (1/4 cup/60 milliliters) 48

SANDWICH SPREADS & SNACKS

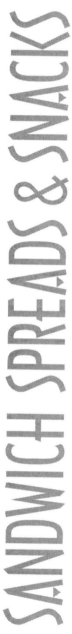

BLUEBERRY PRESERVES
(Strawberry—Raspberry)

1 cup	fresh or frozen blueberries (unsweetened)	250 milliliters
1 teaspoon	lo-cal pectin	5 milliliters
1 teaspoon	sugar replacement	5 milliliters

Place blueberries in top of double boiler. Cook over boiling water until soft and juicy. (Crush berries against sides of double boiler.) Add pectin and sugar replacement. Blend in thoroughly. Cook until medium thick. Preserves can also be made with strawberries or raspberries.

Microwave: Place blueberries in glass bowl. Cook on HIGH for 4 minutes until soft and juicy. (Crush berries against sides of bowl.) Add pectin and sugar. Blend in thoroughly. Cook on HIGH for 30 seconds.

Yield: ⅔ cup (180 milliliters)
Exchange: 1 fruit
Calories: 40

HAMBURGER RELISH

2 quarts	cucumbers (ground)	2 liters
2	onions	2
2	green peppers	2
1	red pepper	1
¼ cup	salt	60 milliliters
2 cups	vinegar	500 milliliters
1 teaspoon	mustard seeds	5 milliliters
1 teaspoon	celery seeds	5 milliliters
1 teaspoon	turmeric	5 milliliters
1 teaspoon	parsley flakes	5 milliliters
2 cups	sugar replacement	500 milliliters

Grind cucumbers, onions, green peppers, and red pepper. Stir in salt. Soak overnight; drain. Combine vinegar, mustard seeds, celery seeds, parsley flakes, and turmeric. Bring to a boil; cook for 10 minutes. Add ground vegetables; cook for 20 minutes. Remove from heat. Add sugar replacement; stir to dissolve. Allow to rest for 24 hours; stir often. Drain slightly if too much liquid accumulates. Pack in scalded jars; seal.

Yield: About 5 pints
Exchange: (1 tablespoon/15 milliliters) Negligible
Calories: (1 tablespoon/15 milliliters) Negligible

BEEF JERKY

2 pounds	flank steak	1 kilogram
¹/₂ cup	soy sauce	125 milligrams
	lemon pepper to taste	
	garlic salt to taste	

Thoroughly chill flank steak. Cut into ¹/₄ x 8-inch (6 x 20-centimeter) strips. Combine soy sauce, lemon pepper, and garlic salt. Marinate steak in sauce for 24 hours; drain. Place on broiler pan. Bake at 150°F (66°C) for 10 to 12 hours, or until dry.

> **Exchange:** (2 strips) 1 high-fat meat
> **Calories:** (2 strips) 108

WRAPPED WIENER

1	wiener	1
³/₈-inch strip	cheese	1-centimeter strip
	dough for 1 biscuit	

Make a thin slit in wiener; insert strip of cheese in slit. Roll or pat biscuit dough thin. Place wiener on edge of dough; roll up. Secure by pinching dough together, or use a toothpick. Bake at 375°F (190°C) for 15 minutes, or until golden brown.

> **Yield:** 1 serving
> **Exchange:** 1¹/₄ meat, 1 bread
> **Calories:** 141

FISH BUNDLES

¹/₂ cup	Herb-Seasoned Stuffing (page 148)	125 milliliters
8 ounces	Cooked Flaked Fish (page 131)	240 grams
1	egg	1

Moisten stuffing with water. Allow to stand 5 minutes, or until soft. (Add extra water if needed.) Blend fish and egg into softened stuffing. Form into 6 patties. Broil for 10 to 15 minutes. Turn once.

> **Yield:** 6 patties
> **Exchange:** (1 patty) 1¹/₄ meat, ¹/₄ bread, ¹/₈ fat
> **Calories:** (1 patty) 45

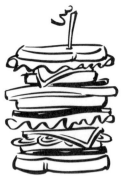

TEENY PIZZA

	dough for 1 biscuit	
1 tablespoon	Tomato Sauce (page 168)	15 milliliters
dash each	garlic powder, oregano, thyme, salt	dash each
¹/₂ ounce	meat of your choice	15 grams
¹/₂ ounce	mozzarella cheese (shredded)	15 grams

Press or roll biscuit dough flat. Roll edge up or place in indivdual baking dish. Combine Tomato Sauce and seasonings. Spread over entire surface of biscuit. Top with meat and cheese. Bake at 450°F (230°C) for 10 minutes.

Yield: 1 serving
Exchange: 1 meat, 1 bread
Calories: 150

GARLIC DILL PICKLES

	firm medium cucumbers (quartered)	
3 cups	water	750 milliliters
3 cups	vinegar	750 milliliters
¹/₂ cup	pickling salt	125 milliliters
1 per jar	dill head	1 per jar
1 per jar	garlic clove	1 per jar

Combine water, vinegar, and pickling salt. Bring to a boil; cook for 5 minutes. Divide cucumbers, dill, and garlic among three scalded 1-quart (1-liter) jars. Fill jars with vinegar mixture. Seal immediately. Ready in 6 to 8 weeks.

Exchange: (1 pickle) Negligible
Calories: (1 pickle) Negligible

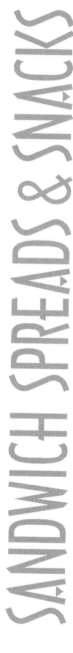

SANDWICH SPREADS & SNACKS

BREAD AND BUTTER PICKLES

4 quarts	cucumbers (sliced)	4 liters
5	onions	5
1 quart	crushed ice	1 liter
1/3 cup	salt	90 milliliters
2 cups	vinegar	500 milliliters
1 1/2 teaspoons	turmeric	7 milliliters
1 1/2 teaspoons	celery seeds	7 milliliters
2 teaspoons	mustard seeds	10 milliliters
1 teaspoon	ginger	5 milliliters
1 1/2 cups	sugar replacement	375 milliliters

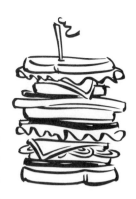

Slice cucumbers and onions; place in large saucepan. Mix ice and salt; stir into cucumbers and onions. Cover. Chill for 5 to 6 hours. Drain; remove ice. Combine vinegar and seasonings. Bring to a boil; simmer for 5 minutes. Add sugar replacement; stir to dissolve. Add drained cucumbers and onions. Bring to a boil. Put into scalded jars and seal.

Yield: 4 to 5 pints
Exchange: (1 tablespoon/15 milliliters) Negligible
Calories: (1 tablespoon/15 milliliters) Negligible

DILL MIDGETS

1 head	dill	1 head
20 to 25	firm midget cucumbers	20 to 25
1/2 teaspoon	alum	2 milliliters
2 teaspoons	pickling salt	10 milliliters
1/2 cup	white vinegar	125 milliliters

Scald 1-pint (1/2-litre) jar. Push dill head to bottom of jar. Fill with midgets. Add alum and pickling salt. Pour vinegar over top. Add enough cold water to fill jar; seal. Shake vigorously. Ready in 8 to 10 weeks.

Yield: 20 to 25 pickles
Exchange: (1 pickle) Negligible
Calories: (1 pickle) Negligible

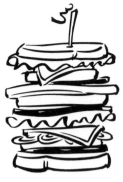

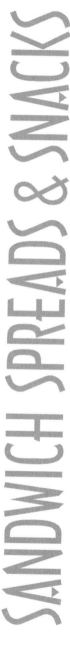

SANDWICH SPREADS & SNACKS

RUSSIAN TEASICLES

2 quarts	water	2 liters
1	cinnamon stick	1
3	whole cloves	3
2 tablespoons	black tea leaves	30 milliliters
6-ounce can	frozen lemon juice (unsweetened)	180-milliliter can
6-ounce can	frozen orange juice	180-milliliter can
1/2 cup	sugar replacement	125 milliliters

Combine water, cinnamon stick, whole cloves, and black tea leaves in large kettle. Bring to a boil; reduce heat and simmer for 15 to 20 minutes. Strain; cool slightly. Add frozen concentrates and sugar replacement. Stir to dissolve. Pour into freezer stick trays; freeze.

Yield: about 38 popsicles
Exchange: (1 popsicle) 1/2 fruit
Calories: (1 popsicle) 5

EGGNOG

1	egg (well beaten)	1
2 teaspoons	sugar replacement	10 milliliters
dash	salt, vanilla extract	dash
3/4 cup	cold milk	180 milliliters
dash	nutmeg to taste	dash

Combine egg with sugar replacement and salt. Add vanilla extract and cold milk. Beat well. Pour into glass or mug; sprinkle with nutmeg.

Yield: 1 serving
Exchange: 1 meat, 1 milk
Calories: 148

PIES & TURNOVERS

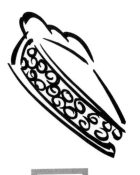

Missing from most discussions of pie is an honest acknowledgment of how high the fat content is. One small slice of a traditional two-crust pie has more than 3 fat exchanges, and that's just the crust. These numbers assume that a standard nine-inch pie is cut into eight slices. If you eat one-sixth of a two-crust pie, you get *four* fat exchanges, again for just the crust portion.

What to do about this depressing pie crust news? We give you many choices in pie crust, ranging from a totally fat-free meringue to a traditional pie crust. It's up to you to decide how many calories and fat exchanges you are willing to spend on pie crust. We're following current standard practice in stating that one serving is one-eighth of a nine-inch pie.

We list the recipes for crusts separate from the recipes for fillings. You decide which crust you wish to pair with which filling. Be sure to combine the calories, exchanges, etc., for the total.

For our meringue pie crust, the crust portion of one slice is only 30 calories. There is no fat or cholesterol, and there are no exchanges. The trade-off is that with a meringue pie crust, you have to plan ahead and give it time to cook and cool, although it is very easy to do. Another trade-off is that a meringue pie crust can be unexciting.

Next best, in terms of fat and calorie scores, is the cottage cheese-based pie crust. One slice of this crust has only 52 calories and 2.8 grams of fat, for half a fat exchange.

Next best is our graham cracker crust. One slice is only 86 calories and 2.2 grams of fat, also half a fat exchange. We made our graham cracker crust with nonfat cream cheese instead of butter or margarine.

Next comes a flour-based pie crust in which we used half margarine and half nonfat cream cheese. One slice of a pie with a bottom crust only has 97 calories and 4.3 grams of fat. It looks beautiful, but we must be honest and tell you that it is not as flaky as Grandmom's pie crust made with (unhealthy) lard.

When we use all margarine for our flour-based pie crust, one slice of bottom-crust-only pie has 140 calories and 8.5 grams of fat. A slice from a pie with a top and bottom crust has 241 calories and 15.5 grams of fat. All these figures are for the crust portion only.

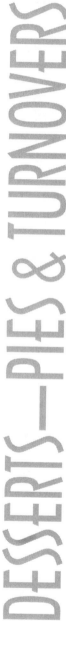

We do have some other crust suggestions. You can use fillo dough to make a nice top crust; the cost per slice is low in calories. We do not recommend using fillo dough for a bottom crust; the dough dissolves into an unattractive goo. The idea of putting a fruit filling into an empty pie pan and then covering it with fillo dough may seem strange when you first hear it. But it works quite will. Our taste testers liked the pies with just a fillo-dough top crust. And it costs almost nothing in calories.

A turnover is like a little pie. We offer a couple of suggestions to get you started. You can substitute any other appropriate filling.

FAT-FREE PIE CRUST

1 cup	egg whites	250 milliliters
1 teaspoon	vanilla extract	5 milliliters
6 packets	concentrated acesulfame-K	6 packets
¹/₄ teaspoon	cream of tartar	1 milliliter
1 tablespoon	sugar	15 milliliters

This is basically an egg-white meringue, so it has very few calories. It's easy to make and looks quite impressive. It's best to make the crust the day before you fill it and serve it. Keep in mind that meringues get sticky in damp weather.

Using an electric mixer, beat the egg whites until foamy, then add the vanilla extract, acesulfame-K, cream of tartar and sugar. Pour the mixture into a 9-inch (23-centimeter) pie pan that has been coated with non-stick cooking spray. Use a spatula to distribute the mixture evenly into a pie crust shape. Bake in a preheated 250°F (120°C) oven for one hour. Turn off the heat and let the pie crust cool in the oven.

Yield:	8 servings	
Exchange:	free	
Each serving:	Calories: 30	Fiber: 0
	Sodium: 86 milligrams	Cholesterol: 0

COTTAGE CHEESE PIE CRUST

¹/₃ cup	flour (sifted)	90 milliliters
2 tablespoons	margarine	30 milliliters
¹/₂ cup	nonfat cottage cheese	125 milliliters

You'll be pleased with this pie crust. It's low-calorie and virtually foolproof.

Drain the cottage cheese dry, then place it in a food processor with a metal blade and blend until pureed. Discard any liquid. Cut the margarine into the dry ingredients as you would for a regular pie crust, then add the cottage cheese, mixing lightly with a fork until a ball of dough is formed. Turn onto a lightly floured pastry cloth and roll it to fit an 8-inch (20-centimeter) or 9-inch (23-centimeter) pie pan coated with nonfat cooking spray. Prick the crust all over with a fork.

Yield:	8 servings	
Exchange:	¹/₂ fat	
Each serving:	Calories: 52	Fiber: trace
	Sodium: 32.3 milligrams	Cholesterol: 1.3 milligrams

BUTTERY GRAHAM CRACKER CRUST

1¹/₄ cups	graham cracker crumbs	310 milliliters
2 ounces	nonfat cream cheese	60 grams
1 teaspoon	butter-flavored extract	5 milliliters
¹/₂ teaspoon	cinnamon	2 milliliters

Using nonfat cream cheese instead of margarine or butter reduces the fat dramatically as compared to the traditional version.

Combine the ingredients in a food processor. Use your fingers or a spoon to press the mixture firmly into a 9-inch (23-centimeter) pie pan. Bake at 325°F (165°C) for 8 to 10 minutes.

Yield:	8 servings	
Exchange:	1 bread	
Each serving:	Calories: 86	Fiber: trace
	Sodium: 133 milligrams	Cholesterol: 3 milligrams

DESSERTS—PIES & TURNOVERS

ONE-CRUST PASTRY PIE CRUST
for a 9-inch (23-centimeter) Shell

1 cup	flour	250 milliliters
3 tablespoons	margarine	45 milliliters
3 tablespoons	nonfat cream cheese	45 milliliters
3 tablespoons	ice water	45 milliliters
1 tablespoon	flour	15 milliliters

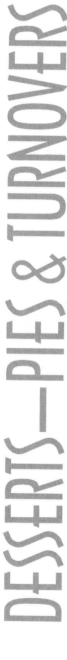

Here we used part margarine and part nonfat cream cheese for a pretty good pie crust. Although it's not as flaky as Grandmom's crust made with (unbelievably) lard, its fat and calorie content are acceptable.

Combine all the ingredients using a pastry blender or process in a food processor for a few seconds. With your hands, firm the dough into a ball. Chill the dough in the refrigerator for at least half an hour.

Sprinkle a small amount of flour on a countertop or a large wooden board. Center the dough on the floured surface. Roll the dough into a circle slightly larger than the pie pan. Carefully lift the pie crust into the pan. If it will be baked unfilled, use a fork to prick the bottom and sides. Bake in a preheated 375°F (190°C) oven for 8 to 9 minutes.

Yield:	8 servings	
Exchange:	1 bread, ½ fat	
Each serving:	Calories: 97	Fiber: trace
	Sodium: 74 milligrams	Cholesterol: trace

TRADITIONAL PIE CRUSTS

Crust for two-crust pie

2 cups	flour	500 milliliters
11 tablespoons	unsalted margarine	165 milliliters
⅓ cup	ice water	90 milliliters

Crust for one-crust pie

1¼ cups	flour	310 milliliters
6 tablespoons	unsalted margarine	90 milliliters
3 tablespoons	ice water	45 milliliters

We decided to include a classic pastry pie crust so you can compare the numbers with the low-fat ones we developed for you. We've included a two-crust pie crust and a one-crust pie crust. Follow the same directions for both.

Put the flour into a bowl. Using two knives or a pastry blender, cut in the margarine until the mixture resembles coarse meal. Add about two tablespoons (30 milliliters) of water and work it gently with a fork. Gradually add and mix in the rest of the water, using your fingers or a pastry blender to work the dough into a ball. Chill the dough for 30 minutes. If you are in a hurry, proceed to the next step immediately. If there is enough dough for two crusts, divide the dough roughly in half and keep half in the refrigerator while you roll the first crust.

On a lightly floured surface, flatten the dough into a circle with roundish edges. Use a rolling pin to roll the dough into a circle slightly bigger than the pie pan, rolling from the center outward. Fold the circle of dough in half and gently lift it onto the pie pan, being careful not to stretch it. Unfold the dough and pat it gently into the pan. Using a kitchen knife, cut off any extra dough that is more than ¾ inch (3 centimeters) beyond the edge of the pan. Fold the outside dough over to make a double thickness of dough around the rim of the pan. Press the dough edge down with a fork, or use your fingers to make a fluted edge. If the crust will be baked without any filling, prick the crust all over with a fork.

Bake in a 425°F (220°C) oven for approximately 12 to 15 minutes or until it is lightly browned.

Yield:	8 servings of crust for two-crust pie
Exchange:	3 fat, 1½ bread
Each serving:	Calories: 241 Fiber: trace
	Sodium: 178 milligrams Cholesterol: 0

GRAHAM CRACKER CRUST
for a 10-inch (25-centimeter) Pie

1½ cups	graham cracker crumbs (18 squares)	375 milliliters
3 packets	concentrated acesulfame-K	3 packets
⅓ cup	margarine or butter (melted)	90 milliliters

This is like the recipe often found on the graham cracker box.

Mix the graham cracker crumbs and acesulfame-K together in a bowl. Add the margarine and mix thoroughly. Press firmly and evenly into the bottom and sides of a pie pan. Bake in a 350°F (175°C) oven for 10 minutes. Cool before adding filling.

Yield:	10 servings
Exchange:	½ bread, 1 fat
Each serving:	Calories: 106 Fiber: trace
	Sodium: 81 milligrams Cholesterol: 0

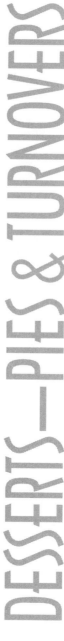

GRAHAM CRACKER CRUST
for an 8-inch (20-centimeter) Pie

1¼ cups	graham cracker crumbs (15 squares)	310 milliliters
2 packets	concentrated acesulfame-K	2 packets
¼ cup	margarine or butter	60 milliliters

Use this recipe for a small pie pan. Follow the previous directions for a 10-inch (25-centimeter) pie.

Yield:	8 servings	
Exchange:	½ bread, 1 fat	
Each serving:	Calories: 106	Fiber: trace
	Sodium: 86 milligrams	Cholesterol: 0

FILLO DOUGH

Greek fillo dough is low in fat and calories and it's easy to use to make pie shells, individual tarts, napoleons, or turnovers. Most grocery stores sell frozen packages. Defrosted dough may be kept in the refrigerator for a few weeks.

To use fillo, bring the dough to room temperature. Arrange two surfaces to work on, one for the current sheet and one to store the balance. Take out sheets of fillo only as needed.

While working on one, be careful to keep the others moist. Fillo dough dries out quickly when uncovered, so have all the equipment and ingredients ready before taking the dough out of the package. Using plastic wrap, cover the sheets you are not currently using. A large, clean, plastic-wastebasket-size bag works better than two narrow sheets of plastic wrap. Place a damp dish towel over the plastic, taking care that the towel does not touch the dough and cause it to fall apart. Discard any problem sheets.

Instructions accompanying fillo suggest covering each layer with softened butter. But using a butter-flavored non-stick cooking spray works well.

Yield:	a sheet of dough is one serving	
Exchange:	2 bread	
Each sheet:	Calories: 180	Fiber: 1 gram
	Sodium: 120 milligrams	Cholesterol: 0

FILLO TOP CRUST
for a 9-inch (23-centimeter) Pie

4 sheets	fillo dough	4 sheets
	butter-flavored non-stick cooking spray	

Fillo dough can be used to make an attractive top crust with few calories and little fat. Put your choice of pie filling into a pie pan with no bottom crust.

Place one large sheet of dough on a dry surface. Spray lightly with non-stick cooking spray. Put a second sheet on top. Place a 9-inch (23-centimeter) metal pie pan face-up in the center of the top layer of the double layer of dough. Spray again. Use scissors to cut away any dough that sticks out more than one inch (2.5 centimeters) around the edge of the pan. Carefully lift this dough up over the top of the filled pie shell. Use scissors to cut off excess dough, more than one inch (2.5 centimeters) around edge. Use your fingers to form the edge into a fluted pie shell. Spray lightly with non-stick cooking spray. Bake in a preheated 375°F (190°C) oven for 7 minutes or until nicely browned.

APPLE PIE FILLING FOR PIE OR TARTS

4 cups	apple (peeled & sliced thin)	1 liter
1 tablespoon	cinnamon	15 milliliters
1 teaspoon	nutmeg	5 milliliters
1 tablespoon	vanilla extract	15 milliliters
2 tablespoons	lemon juice	30 milliliters
6 packets	concentrated acesulfame-K	6 packets
1 teaspoon	grated lemon peel	5 milliliters

The sweetness of the filling depends on the type of apple you choose.

Put the apple slices into a large non-stick pan that has been coated with non-stick cooking spray. Cover and cook for about 10 minutes. Stir occasionally. When the apple slices are soft, add the remaining ingredients and stir to mix.

This recipe makes enough for one 9-inch (23-centimeter) pie or 12 tarts.

Yield:	8 servings	
Exchange:	1½ fruit	
Each serving:	Calories: 89	Fiber: 4 grams
	Sodium: 1 milligram	Cholesterol: 0

DESSERTS—PIES & TURNOVERS

TART SHELLS

Fillo pastry tarts may be available in your supermarket; if not, use this recipe.

Put four sheets of fillo dough on a work surface. Cut a few inches from one side to form squares. Cut each of these squares into four pieces, making 16 small squares.

Take one square and lay it flat. Coat it with non-stick cooking spray. Place another square on top of it, catercorner, forming an eight-pointed star. Carefully press it to the inside or outside of a tart pan or a 6-ounce (180-gram) custard cup that has been sprayed with non-stick cooking spray to make a tart shell that can hold ½ cup (125 milliliters) of filling. Leave the cup in place to protect the delicate shell.

Repeat to make seven other shells. Place them on a cookie sheet, not touching. Bake in a preheated 375°F (190°C) oven for 8 to 9 minutes. When the dough is golden brown, remove turnovers from the oven and let cool for a few minutes. Carefully lift the fillo shells from the custard cups or the tart pans and allow to finish cooling on a wire rack. Before serving, fill with your choice of filling. Good choices include fresh or frozen berries, defrosted (sprinkled with a little aspartame or acesulfame-K, if desired); pudding (vanilla or chocolate, no-sugar, no-fat, instant mixes or other recipes, such as the ones in the pudding chapter); a thin layer of vanilla pudding plus fruit; sugar-free, fat-free frozen yogurt.

These tarts are not good finger food: as they are so thin, they shatter easily. But eaten with a fork or spoon, they are elegant and seem self-indulgent despite their low calories and low fat.

DESSERTS—PIES & TURNOVERS

CREAMY PRUNE PIE FILLING

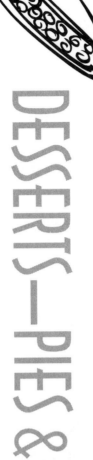

10 packets	concentrated acesulfame-K	10 packets
¹/₃ cup	flour	90 milliliters
pinch	salt (optional)	pinch
2 cups	skim milk	500 milliliters
¹/₃ cup	egg substitute	90 milliliters
1 cup	nonfat sour cream	250 milliliters
1 teaspoon	vanilla extract	5 milliliters
2 teaspoons	grated lemon peel	10 milliliters
1 teaspoon	lemon juice	5 milliliters
¹/₂ cup	pitted prunes (cut into small pieces)	125 milliliters
Topping:		
3	egg whites	3
¹/₄ teaspoon	cream of tartar	1 milliliter
2 teaspoons	sugar	10 milliliters
3 packets	concentrated acesulfame-K	3 packets
¹/₂ teaspoon	cardamom	2 milliliters

The combination of prunes, lemon flavor, and cardamom makes a special "European" dish.

Combine the 10 packets of acesulfame-K, flour, and salt in a saucepan. Add the milk and stir to combine. Bring to a boil and cook for 1 to 2 minutes, stirring with a wire whisk. Turn off the heat. In a separate container, add a small amount of the hot milk and the egg substitute. Return this to the saucepan and cook for several minutes over low heat, stirring with a wire whisk. Let cool for a few minutes. Add the sour cream, vanilla extract, lemon peel, lemon juice, and prune pieces. Whisk together. Pour into a prepared pie shell or into an empty 9-inch (23-centimeter) pan if you wish to reduce calories.

Then prepare the topping. Beat the egg whites with an electric mixer, add in the cream of tartar near the end. Then beat in the sugar, acesulfame-K, and cardamom. Spread the meringue over the top of the pie. Use a rubber spatula to be sure the topping goes all the way to the edges. Bake in a preheated 350°F (175°C) oven for 13 minutes. Cool in the refrigerator.

Yield:	8 servings	
Exchange:	1 milk	
Each serving:	Calories: 97	Fiber: trace
	Sodium: 110 milligrams	Cholesterol: 5 milligrams

DESSERTS—PIES & TURNOVERS

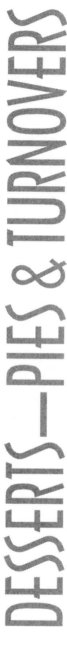

DESSERTS—PIES & TURNOVERS

NOT-QUITE-AMERICAN APPLE (or CHERRY) PIE

4 pieces	fillo dough	4 pieces
4 cups	apple or cherry filling (pages 185 & 189)	1 liter

This is an example of how to combine a dough or crust recipe with a filling recipe.

First make the fruit filling, following the directions on pages 185 or 189. Turn the filling into a 9-inch (23-centimeter) pie pan that has been coated with non-stick vegetable cooking spray. Set aside. Following the general instructions for using fillo dough, spread one sheet of dough onto a work surface and coat it with cooking spray. Spread the second sheet of dough over the first. Spray. Repeat until there are four layers on top of one another. Lift these four layers together and center them over the fruit-filled pie pan. Use a pair of clean scissors to trim away all but one inch (2.5 centimeters) around the edge of the dough. Use your fingers to crimp together the edge to resemble a traditional pie crust. Bake in a preheated 375°F (190°C) oven for 15 minutes or until the top is nicely browned. Watch carefully that it does not overcook.

Yield: 8 servings

APPLE-PRUNE PIE FILLING

1 cup	prunes	250 milliliters
³/₄ cup	apple juice (unsweetened)	190 milliliters
2 teaspoons	finely grated lemon peel	10 milliliters
2 tablespoons	applejack liqueur (optional)	30 milliliters
6	apples (peeled and sliced)	6
1 teaspoon	vanilla extract	5 milliliters
1 teaspoon	lemon juice	5 milliliters
1 teaspoon	cinnamon	5 milliliters
¹/₂ teaspoon	nutmeg	2 milliliters
2 tablespoons	flour	30 milliliters
2 tablespoons	measures-like-sugar saccharin	30 milliliters

You can make a traditional pie by spooning this filling into an unbaked pastry shell and topping it with another crust. To cut way down on fat and calories, spoon the filling into an empty pie pan and top it with a fillo dough crust.

Combine the first four ingredients in a small saucepan; simmer for a few minutes, then turn off the heat. In a separate bowl, combine the apples and the remaining ingredients. Puree the prune mixture in a blender or food processor. Combine with the apple mixture. Spoon into a prepared crust, if desired. Top with a second crust. Bake in a 425°F (220°C) oven for 10 minutes. Turn the heat down to 350°F (175°C) and bake for an additional 40 minutes. Cool on a wire rack.

Yield:	8 servings	
Exchange:	2 fruit	
Each serving:	Calories: 106	Fiber: 4 grams
	Sodium: 2 milligrams	Cholesterol: 0

CHERRY PIE FILLING

2 (14½-ounce) cans	cherries (in water)	2 (411-gram) cans
3 tablespoons	quick-cooking tapioca	45 milliliters
5 packets	concentrated acesulfame-K	5 packets
¼ teaspoon	almond extract	1 milliliter
5 drops	red food coloring	5 drops
1 teaspoon	lemon peel	5 milliliters

Be sure to buy cherries packed in water or juice with no sugar.

Drain the cherries, reserving ⅓ cup (90 milliliters) of the liquid. Whisk together all the remaining ingredients, then let the mixture thicken for 15 minutes. Use a two-crust pastry recipe for the crust or use the fillo recipe below.

To make a cherry pie with a fillo dough crust, follow the general instructions for fillo dough. Spread out one layer and coat it with non-stick cooking spray. Top it with a second layer, and spray. Repeat until there are four layers on top of one another. Lift the dough onto the fruit in the pie pan. Coat with non-stick cooking spray. Use scissors to trim away all but one inch (2.5 centimeters) around the edge. Use your fingers to crimp it in to form an edge. Bake in a preheated 375°F (190°C) oven for 15 minutes.

Yield:	8 servings	
Exchange:	1 fruit	
Each serving:	Calories: 55	Fiber: trace
	Sodium: 1.3 milligrams	Cholesterol: 0

DESSERTS—PIES & TURNOVERS

MARION'S LIME PIE FILLING

1 packet	sugar-free, fat-free lime gelatin	1 packet
⅓ cup	boiling water	90 milliliters
1¼ cups	diet ginger ale	310 milliliters
1 cup	yogurt cheese	250 milliliters
	whipped topping (optional)	

Edith's mother had a friend, Marion, who was famous for her desserts. Some were very complicated; some were very, very easy but tasted so wonderful that everyone assumed Marion spent hours making them. This is our version of Marion's pie. Yogurt cheese is made by letting yogurt drip through cheesecloth overnight in the refrigerator.

Dissolve the gelatin in boiling water in a large bowl, stirring with a large spoon. Add the ginger ale. Stir well to combine. Whisk in the yogurt cheese until blended. The mixture will be thin. Freeze for 10 minutes, then spoon into a prepared pie shell until set. Garnish with whipped topping, if desired.

Yield:	8 servings		
Exchange:	free		
Each serving:	Calories: 19		Fiber: 0
	Sodium: 46 milligrams		Cholesterol: trace

FROZEN RASPBERRY PIE FILLING

1½ cups	sugar-free, reduced-fat vanilla ice cream	375 milliliters
½ cup	raspberries	125 milliliters
1	prepared pie crust	1

This is another of Marion's recipes, modified for diabetic use. It tastes very rich and creamy.

Allow the ice cream to soften at room temperature for approximately an hour; add the raspberries and process until smooth in a food processor. Pour into a pie crust shell. Freeze. Allow the pie to soften for a few minutes at room temperature before serving.

Yield:	8 servings		
Exchange:	½ bread		
Each serving:	Calories: 41		Fiber: trace
	Sodium: 17 milligrams		Cholesterol: 6 milligrams

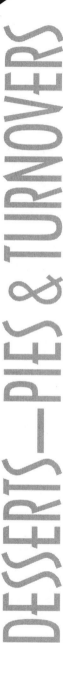

DESSERTS—PIES & TURNOVERS

LEMON CHIFFON PIE FILLING

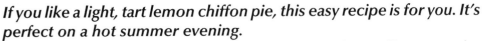

1 packet	unflavored gelatin	1 packet
6 packets	concentrated acesulfame-K	6 packets
4	eggs (separated)	4
¹/₂ cup	lemon juice (fresh is best)	125 milliliters
¹/₄ cup	water	60 milliliters

If you like a light, tart lemon chiffon pie, this easy recipe is for you. It's perfect on a hot summer evening.

Thoroughly mix the gelatin and three packs of acesulfame-K in the top of a double boiler. Beat together the egg yolks, lemon juice, and water; add this to the gelatin.

Cook the mixture over boiling water, stirring constantly until the gelatin is dissolved, about 5 minutes. Remove from the heat. Chill, stirring occasionally until the mixture mounds slightly when dropped from a spoon. Beat the egg whites until stiff. Beat in the remaining acesulfame-K. Fold the gelatin mixture into the stiffly beaten egg whites. Turn into a baked pie shell, if desired. Chill until firm.

Yield:	8 servings
Exchange:	¹/₂ meat
Each serving:	Calories: 46
	Sodium: 38 milligrams

Fiber: trace
Cholesterol: 137 milligrams

QUICK BANANA CREAM PIE FILLING

1	banana (ripe & sliced thin)	1
3 cups	skim milk	750 milliliters
2 packages	sugar-free fat-free vanilla pudding	2 packages

This would be a good project for a cook-in training. You just can't go wrong. Banana cream pie is traditionally served in a flour-based bottom crust.

Place the banana slices in the bottom of the pie shell of your choice. Using an electric mixer, combine the milk and pudding. Pour the mixture over the banana slices. Chill until serving time. Add additional thin slices of banana or whipped topping just before serving, if desired.

Yield:	8 servings
Exchange:	1 bread
Each serving:	Calories: 70
	Sodium: 377 milligrams

Fiber: trace
Cholesterol: 1¹/₂ milligrams

DESSERTS—PIES & TURNOVERS

BLUEBERRY PIE FILLING

12-ounce bag	frozen blueberries	356-gram bag
3 packets	concentrated acesulfame-K	3 packets
1¹/₂ tablespoons	cornstarch dissolved in 2 tablespoons (30 milliliters) water	22 milliliters
¹/₂ teaspoon	vanilla extract	2 milliliters
¹/₂ tablespoon	lemon juice	7 milliliters
¹/₄ teaspoon	cinnamon	1 milliliter

Everyone we know likes blueberry pie. If you can afford the calories and fat exchanges, put this filling between a bottom and top pie crust. If you want a lighter version, put just the filling in an empty pie pan and top it with a fillo crust. This filling is great in a turnover made from fillo dough.

Partially defrost the blueberries at room temperature or in a microwave oven for 60 seconds. Combine all the other ingredients in a saucepan, add the blueberries, and heat over medium heat, stirring constantly until the mixture thickens.

Yield:	8 servings	
Exchange:	¹/₂ fruit	
Each serving:	Calories: 23	Fiber: trace
	Sodium: 2 milligrams	Cholesterol: 0

SHEER DELIGHT PIE FILLING

1 packet	sugar-free, fat-free instant pudding	1 package
1¹/₂ cups	nonfat sour cream	310 milliliters
1 tablespoon	rum extract	15 milliliters
2 tablespoons	measures-like-sugar aspartame	30 milliliters
2 tablespoons	nonfat milk	30 milliliters
1 (8-ounce) can	crushed unsweetened pineapple (in juice, drained)	1 (244-gram) can
¹/₂ cup	flaked coconut	125 milliliters
1	prepared pie shell	1
	banana slices (optional)	
	whipped topping (optional)	

This dessert is rich and delicious, a special-occasion treat. It's great in a baked graham cracker crust.

Combine instant pudding, sour cream, rum extract, aspartame, and milk in a medium bowl. Beat the mixture with a wire whisk until blended and smooth, about a minute, then fold in the pineapple and coconut. Spoon everything into a pie shell. Chill for three hours. Before serving, garnish with sliced bananas or your favorite topping (optional).

Yield:	8 servings	
Exchange:	1 bread, 1 fat, 1 fruit	
Each serving:	Calories: 181	Fiber: 2 grams
	Sodium: 227 milligrams	Cholesterol: 6 milligrams

LUSCIOUS STRAWBERRY PIE FILLING

2 cups	frozen whole strawberries (with no sugar added)	500 millilitres
1 teaspoon	sugar	5 milliliters
1 teaspoon	concentrated aspartame	5 milliliters
1 teaspoon	lemon juice	5 milliliters
1 cup	boiling water	250 milliliters
3-ounce packet	triple berry sugar-free gelatin	8.5 gram packet
2 teaspoons	strawberry extract	10 milliliters
1 pint	sugar-free vanilla nonfat yogurt	500 milliliters
1	prepared pie shell	1

If you can find sugar-free, non-fat frozen yogurt, use it as a base for other flavors. By itself it's a little unexciting, but strawberries bring their own special taste.

Mix the strawberries in a bowl with the sugar, aspartame, and lemon juice. Set aside for approximately an hour. Combine the boiling water and gelatin and stir until completely dissolved. Add the strawberry extract and stir to combine. Add the frozen yogurt and stir until it melts and the mixture is smooth. Freeze for 10 minutes, until the gelatin starts to set. Add the strawberries. Pour into a pie shell of your choice. Refrigerate. Serve when set.

Yield:	8 servings	
Exchange:	1 fruit	
Each serving:	Calories: 58	Fiber: trace
	Sodium: 63 milligrams	Cholesterol: 0

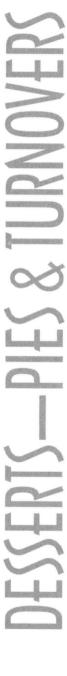

PUMPKIN-APPLE PIE FILLING

¹/₃ cup	unsweetened apple juice	90 milliliters
1 tablespoon	cornstarch	15 milliliters
¹/₂ teaspoon	cinnamon	2 milliliters
1 teaspoon	rum-flavored extract	5 milliliters
3 cups	apples (sliced, cored & peeled) (3 medium or 2 large apples)	750 milliliters
1	egg or equivalent egg substitute	1
³/₄ cup	canned or cooked mashed pumpkin	190 milliliters
¹/₄ teaspoon	ginger	1 milliliter
¹/₂ teaspoon	cinnamon	2 milliliters
¹/₈ teaspoon	cloves	¹/₂ milliliter
¹/₃ cup	measures-like-sugar aspartame	90 milliliters
³/₄ cup	evaporated skim milk	190 milliliters
	sugar-free whipped topping (optional)	

Combine the apple juice, cornstarch, ¹/₂ teaspoon cinnamon, and rum-flavored extract in a large saucepan. Stir constantly. Bring to a boil. Add the apples. Cook for four minutes over medium heat, stirring constantly.

In a mixing bowl, beat the eggs, then add the pumpkin, ginger, cinnamon, cloves, bulk aspartame, and evaporated skim milk. Stir to blend well.

Turn the apple mixture into a 9-inch (23-centimeter) pie shell. Spoon the pumpkin mixture over the apple layer. Bake in a preheated 375°F (190°C) oven for 30 minutes until the pumpkin is set and only slightly browned.

Top with sugar-free whipped topping, if desired.

Yield:	8 servings	
Exchange:	1 bread	
Each serving:	Calories: 132	Fiber: 3 grams
	Sodium: 24 milligrams	Cholesterol: 0

STOVE TOP PUMPKIN PIE FILLING

1¹/₂ cups	cooked or canned pumpkin	375 milliliters
1¹/₂ cups	evaporated nonfat milk	375 milliliters
1 teaspoon	cinnamon	5 milliliters
¹/₂ teaspoon	ginger	2 milliliters
¹/₈ teaspoon	cloves	¹/₂ milliliter
3	eggs (slightly beaten) or equivalent egg substitute	3
1 teaspoon	vanilla extract	5 milliliters
2 teaspoons	rum extract	10 milliliters
20 packets	concentrated acesulfame-K	20 packets
1	prepared pie shell	1
	whipped topping (optional)	

An elegant version of traditional pumpkin pie.

Cook the pumpkin, evaporated milk, cinnamon, ginger, cloves and eggs or egg substitute in the top of a double boiler over hot water, stirring until thick. Cool until the mixture is no longer steaming and add the vanilla and rum extracts and the acesulfame-K.

Beat well, using an electric mixer. Pour into baked pie shell of your choice. Top with sugar-free whipped topping, if desired.

Yield: 8 servings
Exchange: ¹/₂ milk
Each serving: Calories: 68   Fiber: 2 grams
                       Sodium: 51 milligrams   Cholesterol: 0

DESSERTS—PIES & TURNOVERS

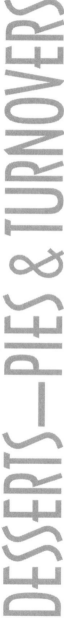
FROZEN CHOCOLATE PIE FILLING

2 cups	sugar-free, reduced-fat chocolate ice cream	500 milliliters
³/₄ cup	diet double fudge soda	190 milliliters
¹/₄ teaspoon	chocolate extract	1 milliliter
1 teaspoon	bulk aspartame	5 milliliters
¹/₄ cup	nonfat ricotta cheese	60 milliliters
1 teaspoon	imitation brandy flavor	5 milliliters

This is a delightful dessert for a summer evening. Try the Graham Cracker Crust recipe (page 183) or use your choice of crust.

Allow the ice cream to soften at room temperature for approximately an hour. Meanwhile, combine the next three ingredients with a wire whisk to make a glaze. Pour into a prebaked graham cracker crust. Freeze. Process the ricotta cheese and brandy flavoring in a food processor until smooth, about a minute. Add the softened ice cream and process until very smooth. Pour into a prepared pie crust.

Yield:	8 servings	
Exchange:	¹/₂ bread	
Each serving:	Calories: 56	Fiber: trace
	Sodium: 28 milligrams	Cholesterol: 8 milligrams

CREAMY MOCHA PIE FILLING

1 packet	unflavored gelatin	1 packet
¹/₂ cup	water	125 milliliters
1 cup	skim milk	250 milliliters
³/₄ cup	fat-free ricotta cheese	190 milliliters
¹/₃ cup	unsweetened cocoa powder	90 milliliters
1 teaspoon	instant coffee granules dissolved in 1 cup (250 millilitres) boiling water	5 milliliters
2 teaspoons	chocolate extract	10 milliliters
10 packets	aspartame	10 packets
	prepared pie shell (see pages 180 to 186)	

This is an easy pie to assemble; we didn't find anyone who didn't like it. It's good in a graham cracker crust.

Combine the gelatin and water in a saucepan; after a few minutes, heat until the gelatin is dissolved. In a blender or food processor, combine the remaining ingredients. Add the dissolved gelatin and blend. Pour into a prepared pie shell and refrigerate.

Yield:	8 servings	
Exchange:	½ milk	
Each serving:	Calories: 33	Fiber: trace
	Sodium: 32 milligrams	Cholesterol: 2.4 milligrams

TURNOVERS

4 sheets	fillo dough	4 sheets
1 cup	filling	250 milliliters

A turnover is a piece of pastry wrapped around a filling, usually fruit-based. When you use fillo dough for the pastry, you get a turnover with a relatively low cost in calories and exchanges, depending of course on the filling you choose. One sheet of fillo dough makes a large turnover. Half would be considered a serving. Fillo dough with fruit filling in it is best eaten on the day it is baked.

Follow the general directions for fillo dough. Spread out one large sheet, coat with butter-flavored non-stick vegetable cooking spray. Fold the dough into thirds the long way. Spray again. Put ¼ cup (60 milliliters) filling on the dough about 2 inches (5 centimeters) from the bottom. Using your fingers, fold the dough up and over the filling; then press down gently. Fold this filled section up towards the plain dough. Fold it up again, as if you were folding a flag. Continue until all the dough has been folded up over the filling. Use your fingers to be sure it is sealed at the edges. Spray the dough again. Put the turnover on a cookie sheet that has been sprayed with non-stick vegetable cooking spray. Repeat with the other three turnovers, or as many as you want. Bake in a preheated 375°F (190°C) oven for 10 minutes.

Yield:	4 turnovers (filling counted separately)	
Exchange:	1 bread	
Each turnover:	Calories: 72	Fiber: trace
	Sodium: 120 milligrams	Cholesterol: 0

DESSERTS—PIES & TURNOVERS

APPLE TURNOVERS

2 slices	bread (crust removed)	2 slices
1	apple (peeled, cored & sliced thin)	1
1 teaspoon	lemon juice	5 milliliters
¹/₄ teaspoon	cinnamon	1 milliliter
1 packet	concentrated acesulfame-K	1 packet

Need something to serve in a pinch? These turnovers can be made in only 10 minutes and are quite tasty.

Roll the bread thin with a rolling pin. Microwave the other ingredients until the apple is tender. The length of time will depend on the type of apple and the power of the oven. Start with 10 seconds on medium and adjust from there. The key is, you don't want the apple mushy. Place half the mixture on each piece of bread. Fold the bread diagonally to form a triangle. Moisten the edges of the bread and press the sides of the turnover together with a fork. Lightly spray both sides with vegetable cooking spray. Place on a cookie sheet coated with non-stick vegetable cooking spray. Bake at 425°F (220°C) for about 7 minutes or until brown.

Yield:	2 turnovers	
Exchange:	1 bread, ¹/₂ fruit	
Each turnover:	Calories: 95	Fiber: 2 grams
	Sodium: 102 milligrams	Cholesterol: 1 milligram

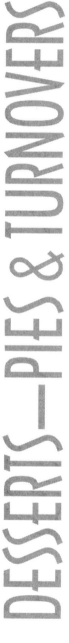

DESSERTS—PIES & TURNOVERS

CAKES, TORTES, & CAKE ROLLS

Making "diabetic" cakes is a challenge; we offer you some tips here. Because sugar is needed to add lightness and a tender texture, it cannot be eliminated completely. We use a bare minimum of sugar and then bolster the sweet taste with artificial sweeteners. We substitute some new no-fat products, such as nonfat sour cream, yogurt, buttermilk, mayonnaise, cream cheese, etc. We offer a few other hints on making "diabetic" cakes.

• Watch cakes carefully near the end of the baking time. Low-sugar, low-fat cakes can easily overcook. Set your timer for the minimum time, then test for doneness. With most cakes, a toothpick inserted in the middle should come out clean.

• Use lots of beaten egg whites to add a light touch; using a minimum amount of sugar and fat can lead to a dense texture. You may want to save the unwanted egg yolks as "pet" food; animals don't suffer from cholesterol problems as some humans do.

• It often works well to use cake flour rather than regular flour. This too lightens a low-sugar, low-fat product.

• Bake cakes in fairly small containers to minimize the amount of time needed for baking. In larger pans, cakes with only egg whites can become rubbery. Cupcake pans work well, as do small loaf pans.

• Slice leftover cake and freeze the individual slices well wrapped. That way you can defrost just the right amount. Do not expect low-sugar, low-fat cakes to remain fresh for a long time. Freezing works well. Take a few strawberries or raspberries out of a freezer bag and serve them with a defrosted cake slice.

• A person with a sweet tooth may want a little extra sweetness. As soon as a cake is out of the oven, poke a few holes in the top with a fork and drizzle in aspartame dissolved in an equal amount of water. Cupcakes can be rolled in the dissolved aspartame.

Making frosting is another real challenge since traditional frostings are basically mixtures of sugar and fat. The challenge is to make something that tastes good. A combination of artificial sweetener, cornstarch, and nonfat dry milk may look like frosting but the taste is disappointing. Our frosting recipes, based on ingredients such as nonfat cream cheese, are quite tasty. But to be honest, plan to serve the cake within a few hours of frosting it. These frostings do not have the staying power of sugary, fatty frostings. You can eliminate frosting by serving a slice of cake with a small amount of unsweetened applesauce; try adding a little cinnamon and aspartame.

Our frosting recipes give the number of calories, exchanges, etc., per tablespoon. That way you can figure according to how many tablespoons (milliliters) you are eating.

DESSERTS—CAKES

GINGERBREAD

1 cup	flour	250 milliliters
³/₄ teaspoon	baking soda	4 milliliters
1 teaspoon	cinnamon	5 milliliters
¹/₂ teaspoon	dry mustard	2 milliliters
1 teaspoon	ginger	5 milliliters
dash	salt (optional)	dash
2 tablespoons	nonfat yogurt	30 milliliters
2 tablespoons	melted margarine or butter	30 milliliters
¹/₄ cup	molasses	60 milliliters
6 packets	concentrated acesulfame-K	6 packets
2 tablespoons	Prune Puree (pages 206 to 207)	30 milliliters
3	egg whites	3
Glaze Ingredients:		
2 tablespoons	hot water	30 millilitres
2 teaspoons	measures-like-sugar aspartame	10 millilitres
¹/₂ teaspoon	lemon extract	2 millilitres

This cake looks ordinary, but the taste is quite special. If you want to add something on top, try our Lemon Sauce or an appropriate whipped topping.

Sift together the flour, baking soda, cinnamon, mustard, ginger, and salt. Set aside. In a separate bowl, whisk together the yogurt, margarine, molasses, acesulfame-K, and prune puree. Add the flour-and-spice mixture to the wet mixture and stir together. In a separate bowl, beat the egg whites until stiff. Gradually beat the beaten egg whites into the batter. Pour the batter into an 8-inch (20-centimeter) round pan that has been sprayed with non-stick vegetable cooking spray. Bake in a preheated 325°F (165°C) oven for 20 to 25 minutes or until a toothpick comes out clean. As soon as the gingerbread is out of the oven, combine the glaze ingredients. Use a toothpick to poke holes in the top of the gingerbread. Then use a pastry brush to brush the glaze over the top.

Yield:	10 servings	
Exchange:	1 bread	
Each serving:	Calories: 89	Fiber: 0.4 grams
	Sodium: 130 milligrams	Cholesterol: 0

ANGEL FOOD CAKE

1 cup	flour	250 milliliters
¹/₄ cup	sugar	60 milliliters
3 packets	concentrated acesulfame-K	3 packets
1¹/₂ cups	egg whites (12)	375 milliliters
1¹/₂ teaspoons	cream of tartar	7 milliliters
¹/₄ teaspoon	salt	1 milliliter
¹/₄ cup	sugar	60 milliliters
4 packets	concentrated acesulfame-K	4 packets
1¹/₂ teaspoons	vanilla extract	7 milliliters
¹/₂ teaspoon	almond extract	2 milliliters

Did you know that you should "break" angel food cake apart instead of using a knife to slice it? With a knife you compress the cake. Instead, use a special slicer or take two forks (one in each hand), and starting with the inside hole, jab the tines into the cake, keeping the forks very close together. Then work a line across to the outside by tearing the cake as you gently separate the forks.

Sift together the flour, first amount of sugar, and first amount of acesulfame-K. Set aside. In a large mixing bowl, combine the egg whites, cream of tartar, and salt. With an electric mixer, beat until foamy. Mix together the second amount of sugar and the second acesulfame-K. Gradually add this mixture, a tablespoon (15 milliliters) at a time, to the egg whites. Continue beating until stiff peaks form. Fold in the vanilla and almond extracts. Sprinkle the flour mixture over the beaten egg whites. Fold gently just until the flour disappears. Fold the matter into an ungreased 10 x 4-inch (25 x 10-centimeter) tube pan.

Bake in a 375°F (190°C) oven for 30 to 35 minutes, until no imprint remains after finger lightly touches the top of the cake. The top should be golden brown. To cool, turn the baked cake over. For best results stand the tube pan on a custard cup or put a bottle in the center hole to hold the top away from the counter so circulation will occur. Remove the cake from the pan only after it is thoroughly cool. Drizzle with bittersweet topping, fruit topping, or sliced fresh fruit.

Yield:	24 slices	
Exchange:	¹/₂ bread	
Each slice:	Calories: 42	Fiber: 1 gram
	Sodium: 178 milligrams	Cholesterol: 0.7 milligrams

DESSERTS—CAKES

BOSTON CREAM PIE

2 cups	cake flour	500 milliliters
1 tablespoon	baking powder	15 milliliters
1/4 teaspoon	salt (optional)	1 milliliter
1 cup	egg substitute	250 milliliters
1/3 cup	sugar	90 milliliters
6 packets	concentrated saccharin	6 packets
1 1/2 teaspoons	vanilla extract	7 milliliters
1/2 teaspoon	butter-flavored extract	2 milliliters
1/3 cup	canola oil	90 milliliters
1 cup	egg whites (at room temperature)	250 milliliters
1/2 teaspoon	cream of tartar	2 milliliters

Cream Filling:

1 1/2 cups	skim milk	375 milliliters
1 package	fat-free, sugar-free vanilla instant pudding	1 package

Chocolate Topping:

1/2	cream filling (above)	1/2
1 tablespoon	cocoa	15 milliliters

No one will ever guess this is a diabetic dessert. Your guests will be impressed.

Sift together the flour, baking powder, and salt. Set aside. In a separate bowl, beat the egg substitute until light and fluffy. Add the sugar, saccharin, vanilla and butter extracts. Add the oil. Add the flour mixture. In another bowl, beat the egg whites until thick. Add the cream of tartar and continue beating until stiff. Stir about one-third of the stiff egg whites into the flour mixture to lighten. Then fold in the remaining egg whites. Pour into two 8-inch (20-centimeter) cake pans that have been coated with non-stick cooking spray. Bake in a preheated 350°F (175°C) oven for 25 minutes or until done.

Cream Filling: Mix together the milk and pudding mix until thick. Spread half the cream filling between the layers.

Chocolate Topping: Combine the other half of the cream filling with cocoa. Spread on top of the cream pie.

Yield:	12 servings
Exchange:	1 bread, 1 milk
Each servings:	Calories: 172
	Sodium: 63 milligrams

Fiber: 0.5 grams
Cholesterol: 0.5 milligrams

RICH CHOCOLATE CAKE

1¹/₃ cups	cake flour	340 milliliters
¹/₃ cup	unsweetened cocoa powder	90 milliliters
¹/₄ teaspoon	baking powder	1 milliliter
¹/₄ teaspoon	baking soda	1 milliliter
pinch	salt (optional)	pinch
¹/₂ cup	egg substitute	125 milliliters
1 teaspoon	vanilla extract	5 milliliters
1 tablespoon	raspberry liqueur	15 milliliters
¹/₂ cup	nonfat buttermilk	125 milliliters
4 tablespoons	margarine or butter	60 milliliters
2 tablespoons	Prune Puree (pages 206 to 207)	30 milliliters
15 packets	concentrated acesulfame-K	15 packets
3 tablespoons	sugar	45 milliliters
6	egg whites	6
¹/₄ teaspoon	cream of tartar	1 millilitre
¹/₂ cup	frozen raspberries	125 milliliters
¹/₂ teaspoon	concentrated aspartame	2 milliliters

Don't let the long list of ingredients intimidate you; this cake is worth the effort!

Sift the first five ingredients together twice; set aside. Combine the egg substitute and vanilla extract, raspberry liqueur, and buttermilk. Using an electric mixer, cream the margarine or butter and the prune puree. Add acesulfame-K and sugar and beat well. Gradually add the egg substitute alternately with the flour mixture. Beat until well combined. Beat the egg whites until stiff. Add the cream of tartar and continue beating. Add a small amount of egg whites to the batter to lighten it. With a rubber spatula, fold in the remaining beaten whites. Pour into two 8-inch (20-centimeter) round cake pans that have been coated with non-stick cooking spray. Bake in a preheated 350°F (175°C) oven for 30 to 35 minutes. Cool, then invert onto a plate. Combine the raspberries and aspartame in a food processor to make raspberry puree. Spread raspberry puree over the top of one layer. Put the other layer on top and cover with raspberry puree.

Decorate top with whole raspberries if desired.

Yield:	10 servings	
Exchange:	2 bread, ¹/₂ fat	
Each serving:	Calories: 189	Fiber: 1.74 grams
	Sodium: 90 milligrams	Cholesterol: 0

DESSERTS—CAKES

APPLESAUCE-CARROT CAKE

2 cups	flour	500 milliliters
2 teaspoons	baking powder	10 milliliters
2 teaspoons	baking soda	10 milliliters
1 tablespoon	cinnamon	15 milliliters
1 teaspoon	allspice	5 milliliters
1 teaspoon	nutmeg	5 milliliters
1/2 cup	pineapple (canned & crushed)	125 milliliters
1/4 cup	raisins	60 milliliters
1/2 cup	walnuts (chopped)	125 milliliters
1/4 cup	sugar	60 milliliters
3 packets	concentrated acesulfame-K	3 packets
3/4 cup	egg substitute or 3 eggs	190 milliliters
1/2 cup	measures-like-sugar saccharin	125 milliliters
1/2 cup	nonfat sour cream	125 milliliters
1/2 cup	unsweetened applesauce	125 milliliters
2 teaspoons	vanilla extract	10 milliliters
2 cups	shredded carrots	500 milliliters
2/3 cup	shredded coconut (optional)	180 milliliters

Carrot cakes tend to be very high in fat because of the large amount of oil used. This recipe gets its moist good taste from pineapple, apple- sauce, and nonfat sour cream. It has a wonderful texture and tastes very rich.

Sift together the flour, baking powder, baking soda, and spices. In a blender or food processor, blend the pineapple, raisins, nuts, and sugar. Do not liquefy. Mix together the acesulfame-K, eggs, saccharin, sour cream, applesauce, vanilla, and the blender mixture. Beat well. Add the flour mixture. Mix well. Add the carrots and coconut. Stir gently. Pour into a 10-inch (25-centimeter) cake pan coated with non-stick cooking spray. Bake at 350°F (175°C) for 50 to 60 minutes or until a cake tester inserted into the center comes out clean. Cool in the pan on a cooling rack. Remove from the pan and cut horizontally to make a two-layer cake. Frost between the layers and on top with Applesauce-Carrot Cake Frosting (recipe follows).

Yield:	12 servings	
Exchange:	2 bread	
Each serving:	Calories: 165	Fiber: 1.6 grams
	Sodium: 304 milligrams	Cholesterol: 1.3 milligrams

APPLESAUCE-CARROT CAKE FROSTING

8 ounces	nonfat cream cheese (softened)	240 milliliters
¹/₂ cup	bulk aspartame	125 milliliters
1 teaspoon	lemon extract	5 milliliters
1 teaspoon	butter-flavored extract	5 milliliters

Although this is a variation of the classic carrot cake frosting, you might want to try it on other flavorful cakes as well.

Beat all ingredients together until smooth.

Yield:	12 tablespoons	
Exchange:	free	
1 Tablespoon:	Calories: 17	Fiber: 0
(15 millilitres)	Sodium: 90 milligrams	Cholesterol: 2.7 milligrams

SHORTCAKE

1³/₄ cup	flour	340 milliliters
1 teaspoon	sugar	5 milliliters
3 packets	concentrated acesulfame-K	3 packets
2 teaspoons	baking powder	10 milliliters
¹/₂ teaspoon	baking soda	2 milliliters
dash	salt (optional)	dash
3 tablespoons	margarine or butter	45 milliliters
⁵/₈ cup	nonfat milk or nonfat buttermilk	150 milliliters

People who like genuine shortcake with their strawberries or peaches will love this! Of course, others enjoy angel cake as a base for sweetened fruit. Those who wish to cut back on calories or exchanges can spoon fruit over half a shortcake.

Combine the flour, sugar, acesulfame-K, baking powder, baking soda, and salt. Cut in the margarine. Using a food processor makes this very quick and easy. Then add the milk and process, or use your hands to gather the dough into a ball.

Put the dough on a lightly floured surface. Work it briefly into a ball and then flatten it. Use a rolling pin to flatten it out; the dough should be about ³/₄ inch (1.75 centimeters) thick. Use a round biscuit cutter to cut out 10 circles. Place the biscuits on a baking sheet. Bake in a preheated 450°F (230°C) oven for 8 to 9 minutes, until lightly brown.

To serve, halve each biscuit and serve with fruit and whipped topping, if desired.

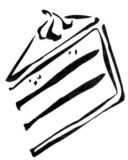

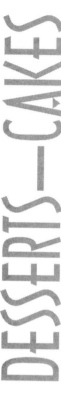

DESSERTS—CAKES

Yield:	10 servings	
Exchange:	1 bread, ¹/₂ fat	
Each serving:	Calories: 111	Fiber: trace
	Sodium: 103 milligrams	Cholesterol: trace

HOT-MILK SPONGE CAKE

1 cup	sifted cake flour	250 milliliters
1 teaspoon	baking powder	5 milliliters
3	eggs	3
¹/₄ cup	sugar	60 milliliters
3 packets	concentrated acesulfame-K	3 packets
¹/₄ cup	hot milk	60 milliliters
1 teaspoon	vanilla extract	5 milliliters
	fruit (optional)	
	whipped topping (optional)	

Grease two 8-inch (20-centimeter) round layer-cake pans. Dust lightly with flour and baking powder mixed together. Using an electric mixer at high speed, beat the eggs in a small, deep bowl until they are light and fluffy; slowly beat in the sugar and acesulfame-K until the mixture is almost double in volume and is very thick. Turn the speed to low; beat in the hot milk and vanilla. Fold in the flour mixture, a third at a time, until just blended. Pour into the prepared pan.

Bake in a 350°F (175°C) oven for 15 to 20 minutes or until the centers spring back when lightly pressed with a fingertip. Cool in the pans on wire racks for 10 minutes. Then loosen cakes carefully around the edges with a knife, turn out onto the wire racks, and cool completely. To serve, put fresh fruit (or well-drained canned fruit packed in its own unsweetened juice) and your favorite whipped topping between the two layers and on top of the cake.

Yield:	8 servings	
Exchange:	1 bread	
Each serving:	Calories: 108	Fiber: 0
	Sodium: 79 milligrams	Cholesterol: 103 milligrams

PRUNE PUREE
(as Fat Replacement)

1 cup	pitted prunes	250 milliliters
¹/₄ cup	unsweetened apple juice	60 milliliters
1 tablespoon	flavoring (vanilla extract or lemon extract or liqueur)	15 milliliters

Use a food processor to puree all the ingredients. Store the mixture in the refrigerator. Use it as a fat substitute in cooking.

Yield: 1¼ cup (310 milliliters)   **Exchange:** free
¼ cup (60 milliliters) contains:
Calories: 13   Fiber: 0.45 grams
Sodium: 0.4 milligrams   Cholesterol: 0

CHEESECAKES

The new nonfat dairy products make it easy to make cheesecakes that fit into diabetic meal plans. These products also add calcium and protein. Here are a few hints about using these new nonfat products.

Nonfat ricotta cheese
Check the dates on the label before you buy; use the cheese while it's still fresh. Nonfat ricotta is used not only in cooking, it also makes a nice (and fat-free) spread for toast and other foods; try it with a little added nutmeg and aspartame.

Nonfat cottage cheese
Process in a food processor or blender for a full two to three minutes to eliminate the curds before using in cooking.

Nonfat cream cheese
Microwave for 30 seconds to soften before adding it to a recipe.

Yogurt
Don't be misled by clever labels. Be sure the yogurt is 100% nonfat. It should also be free of sugar and other caloric sweeteners such as fruit purees. Some yogurts are sweetened with only aspartame or Nutra-Sweet.

Skim Milk
Skim milk does not create rich, creamy desserts the way cream does, although it's fairly innocuous. So add a little cornstarch dissolved in water to thicken dishes made with skim milk. Opinions vary on the use of canned evaporated skim milk. Some people like it when it is disguised by tasty ingredients. One friend, however, refers to it as the kiss of death to any recipe's chances of tasting good.

Egg substitutes
These are a popular way to avoid cholesterol and are more convenient to use in cooking than whole eggs. Egg substitutes can be found in supermarkets either chilled near the eggs or frozen in the freezer section. Some egg substitutes are totally non-fat, others have a very small amount of fat. We had more success cooking with a defrosted egg substitute that has a tiny amount of corn oil than with the totally fat-free versions.

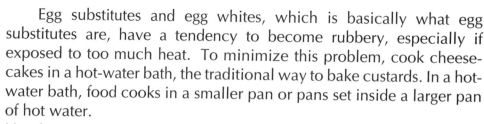
Egg substitutes and egg whites, which is basically what egg substitutes are, have a tendency to become rubbery, especially if exposed to too much heat. To minimize this problem, cook cheesecakes in a hot-water bath, the traditional way to bake custards. In a hot-water bath, food cooks in a smaller pan or pans set inside a larger pan of hot water.

Here's an easy way to manage: Preheat the oven, open the oven door, and slide the lower oven rack partway out. Set the larger pan on this rack. Put the smaller pan(s) of uncooked food in the center of the larger pan. Take a teakettle of boiling water and very carefully pour boiling water into the larger pan. Be sure you do not spill or splatter any water inside the smaller pan. Also, if you're using a springform pan, which is great for cheesecake, be sure the rim is tightly attached to the bottom rim.

Gelatin in cheesecake

Opinions vary on this subject. Some people declare vehemently that "real" cheesecake does not have gelatin. Others like gelatin-based desserts.

Crust

As far as crusts are concerned, you can decide for yourself. Some people like a graham cracker crust, which is described on page 183. To save calories, many cheesecake recipes suggest you simply sprinkle a few tablespoons of graham cracker crumbs on the base of the pan. Of course, you can make a cheesecake with no crust or bottom layer.

GRANOLA TOPPING

3 cups	oatmeal	750 milliliters
¹/₂ cup	wheat germ	125 milliliters
²/₃ cup	sliced unsalted almonds (optional)	180 milliliters
1 tablespoon	safflower oil	15 milliliters
2 tablespoons	molasses	30 milliliters
¹/₂ cup	unsweetened apple juice	125 milliliters

If you like a crunchy topping on frozen yogurt or other desserts, make up some granola topping and keep it on hand.

Mix the oatmeal, wheat germ, and almonds in a lasagna or jelly-roll pan. Heat the remaining ingredients in a saucepan and stir to combine. Drizzle this over the oatmeal mixture, using a spatula to push the mixture around in the pan until evenly coated. Bake in a 325°F (165°C) oven for about 30 minutes. Then mix again and bake for an additional 10 minutes. The longer you cook it, the crunchier the granola gets.

Makes 4¹/₂ cups (1¹/₈ liters).

	Yield:	70 tablespoons (1¹/₈ liters)	
	Exchange:	free	
1 tablespoon:		Calories: 12	Fiber: trace
(15 milliliters)		Sodium: 16 milligrams	Cholesterol: 0

HEALTHFUL CHEESECAKE

¹/₄ cup	graham cracker crumbs	60 milliliters
2 cups	yogurt cheese (see note below)	500 milliliters
2 teaspoons	vanilla extract	10 milliliters
¹/₂ cup	egg substitute	125 milliliters
2 tablespoons	cornstarch	30 milliliters
6 packets	concentrated acesulfame-K	6 packets

Topping:

¹/₂ cup	nonfat sour cream	125 milliliters
2 teaspoons	sugar	10 milliliters
2 teaspoons	concentrated acesulfame-K	10 milliliters
1 teaspoon	vanilla extract	5 milliliters

This is a healthy version of the old-fashioned cheesecake everyone loves. We don't think you'll miss the fat!

Spray a 9-inch (23-centimeter) springform (or other) pie pan with non-stick cooking spray. Sprinkle it evenly with graham-cracker crumbs. Set aside.

Use an electric mixer to combine the next five ingredients. Beat until creamy. Pour the mixture onto the crumbs. Bake in a preheated 325°F (165°C) oven for 35 minutes. Remove from the oven and let cool. Refrigerate. Combine the topping ingredients and pour the mixture over the baked, chilled cheesecake. Return it to the oven for 10 minutes. Chill. Run a knife around the edge of the pan to loosen the cheesecake.

	Yield:	12 servings	
	Exchange:	¹/₂ bread	
Each serving:		Calories: 49	Fiber: trace
		Sodium: 68 milligrams	Cholesterol: 2 milligrams

Note: Yogurt cheese is made by letting yogurt drip through cheesecloth overnight in the refrigerator.

APPLE CHEESECAKE

1 pound	nonfat cottage cheese	480 grams
²/₃ cup	nonfat sour cream	180 milliliters
4 teaspoons	fructose	20 milliliters
2	eggs	2
1 tablespoon	all-purpose flour	15 milliliters
¹/₂ teaspoon	nutmeg	2 milliliters
pinch	cinnamon	pinch
1	juice of one lemon	1
4	small apples (peeled, cored & sliced into half moons)	4
	Graham-Cracker Crust (page 183)	

This cheesecake is fabulous. Some people like to pour the batter into a prebaked graham cracker crust.

Beat the cottage cheese, sour cream, fructose, eggs, flour, nutmeg, and cinnamon until smooth. Stir in the lemon juice. Spread half the apples in the bottom, over a crust if you like. Pour the cottage cheese mixture over the apples. Top with the remaining apples. Bake in a preheated oven at 375°F (190°C) or until set. Cool completely.

Yield:	10 servings	
Exchange:	1 bread	
Each serving:	Calories: 101	Fiber: 1.1 grams
	Sodium: 36 milligrams	Cholesterol: 61 milligrams

CHEESECAKE WITH JELLY GLAZE

8 ounces	nonfat cream cheese	250 milliliters
1 cup	nonfat yogurt (sweetened with aspartame)	250 milliliters
1 package	unsweetened gelatin	1 package
¹/₄ cup	water	60 milliliters
1 tablespoon	measures-like-sugar aspartame	15 milliliters
1 cup	fresh fruit (cut into pieces) or canned (no sugar added)	250 milliliters
3 tablespoons	jelly (made with saccharin)	45 milliliters

This looks more like a pie than a cheesecake, but it tastes like a cheesecake. The top looks lovely with slices of kiwi and raspberry or strawberry halves.

Combine the cream cheese and yogurt and beat until smooth. In a small saucepan, sprinkle the gelatin into the water; let soften for 2 minutes. Over low heat, stir to dissolve the gelatin. Remove from the heat and add to cream cheese mixture. Add the aspartame. With an electric mixer, beat until smooth. Pour into a crust of your choice (A graham-cracker crust is traditional.) Arrange the fruit on top. Microwave the jelly for 30 seconds or heat in a saucepan over low heat. When jelly is liquefied, use a pastry brush to glaze the top of the pie.

Yield:	8 servings	
Exchange:	1 milk	
Each serving:	Calories: 60	Fiber: ¹/₂ gram
	Sodium: 164 milligrams	Cholesterol: 4 milligrams

GRANOLA CHEESECAKE

Crust:

¹/₄ **cup**	margarine or butter (melted)	60 milliliters
1 tablespoon	water	15 milliliters
3 packets	concentrated acesulfame-K	3 packets
1 cup	Granola Topping (page 208)	250 milliliters

Filling:

8 ounces	nonfat cream cheese (softened)	250 milliliters
1 cup	nonfat cottage cheese (drained)	250 milliliters
¹/₂ **cup**	egg substitute or 2 eggs	125 milliliters
3 packets	concentrated acesulfame-K	3 packets
1 teaspoon	vanilla extract	5 milliliters
1 tablespoon	flour	15 milliliters

Topping:

¹/₃ **cup**	Granola Topping (page 208)	90 milliliters

A super combination—creamy cheesecake with a crunch.

Stir the crust ingredients together and press the mixture into the bottom of a 9-inch (23-centimeter) springform pan. Set aside. Beat the filling ingredients together until smooth. Spoon this carefully over the crust. Sprinkle the top with granola topping. Bake in a 375°F (190°C) oven for 40 minutes or until set. Cool before removing cake from the pan.

Yield:	10 servings	
Exchange:	1 meat	
Each serving:	Calories: 88	Fiber: trace
	Sodium: 186 milligrams	Cholesterol: 5.2 milligrams

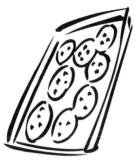

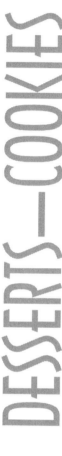

CHOCOLATE-NUT REFRIGERATOR COOKIES

¹/₄ cup	shortening	60 milliliters
1 tablespoon	granulated brown sugar replacement	15 milliliters
1	egg	1
1-ounce square	unsweetened chocolate (melted)	30-gram square
¹/₂ teaspoon	vanilla extract	2 milliliters
2 tablespoons	walnuts (finely ground)	30 milliliters
2 tablespoons	sour milk	30 milliliters
1 tablespoon	water	15 milliliters
1 cup	flour	250 milliliters
1 teaspoon	baking powder	5 milliliters
dash	salt	dash

Cream together shortening and brown sugar replacement. Add egg; beat well. Add melted chocolate, vanilla, walnuts, sour milk and water; beat to mix thoroughly. Add flour, baking powder and salt, and beat to blend. Shape into a roll, 1¹/₂ inches (3³/₄ centimeters) in diameter. Wrap in plastic wrap or waxed paper. Refrigerate at least 2 hours or overnight. Cut into ¹/₄-inch (6-millimeter)-thick slices and place on ungreased cookie sheet. Bake at 400°F (200°C) for 8 to 10 minutes.

Microwave: Place 6 to 8 cookies on waxed paper. Cook on LOW for 3 to 4 minutes, or until tops are set. Cool.

Yield: 30 cookies
Exchange: (1 cookie) ¹/₂ vegetable, ¹/₂ fat
Calories: (1 cookie) 33

TEATIME PUFFS

2	egg whites	2
¹/₄ teaspoon	salt	1 milliliter
2 tablespoons	granulated sugar replacement	30 milliliters
¹/₂ cup	creamy peanut butter (softened)	125 milliliters

Beat egg whites and salt until frothy. Add sugar replacement, beating until mixture is stiff, and fold in peanut butter. Drop by teaspoonfuls onto lightly greased cookie sheets. Bake at 325°F (165°C) for 20 minutes.

Yield: 24 cookies
Exchange: (2 cookies) ¹/₂ medium-fat meat, ¹/₂ fat
Calories: (2 cookies) 64

CREAM CHEESE COOKIES

¼ **cup**	vegetable shortening	60 milliliters
¼ **cup**	cream cheese (softened)	60 milliliters
2 teaspoons	granulated fructose	10 milliliters
1 teaspoon	granulated sugar replacement	5 milliliters
1	egg	1
1 tablespoon	water	15 milliliters
1 cup	flour	250 milliliters
½ **teaspoon**	baking powder	2 milliliters
dash	salt	dash

Cream together shortening, cream cheese, fructose and sugar replacement. Add egg and water, beating well. Sift together flour, baking powder and salt, and add to creamed mixture. Mix until thoroughly blended. Shape into a roll, 1½ inches (3¾ centimeters) in diameter. Refrigerate at least 2 hours or overnight. Cut into thin slices and place on ungreased cookie sheets. Bake at 350°F (175°C) for 8 to 10 minutes.

Yield: 30 cookies
Exchange: (2 cookies) ½ fruit, ½ fat
Calories: (2 cookies) 74

WALNUT MACAROONS

2 cups	quick-cook rolled oats (uncooked)	500 milliliters
2 tablespoons	granulated sugar replacement	30 milliliters
¼ **teaspoon**	salt	1 milliliter
2 teaspoons	vanilla extract	10 milliliters
½ **cup**	liquid shortening	125 milliliters
1	egg (well beaten)	1
½ **cup**	walnuts (very finely chopped)	125 milliliters

Combine oats, sugar replacement, salt, vanilla and liquid shortening in medium mixing bowl. Stir to mix well. Cover and refrigerate overnight. Add beaten egg and chopped walnuts and stir to blend thoroughly. Pack a small amount of cookie mixture level into teaspoon. Pat out onto ungreased cookie sheet. Bake at 350°F (175°C) for 15 minutes.

Microwave: Place 6 to 8 cookies in circle on waxed paper. Cook on LOW for 4 to 5 minutes.

Yield: 42 cookies
Exchange: (1 cookie) 1 fat
Calories: (1 cookie) 40

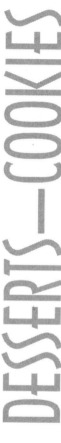

PEANUT-BUTTER COOKIES

¹/₄ **cup**	margarine	60 milliliters
¹/₄ **cup**	creamy peanut butter	60 milliliters
2 tablespoons	granulated brown sugar replacement	30 milliliters
1 tablespoon	granulated sugar replacement	15 milliliters
1	egg	1
¹/₄ **cup**	water	60 milliliters
1 teaspoon	vanilla extract	5 milliliters
1¹/₂ cups	flour	375 milliliters
1 teaspoon	baking soda	5 milliliters
¹/₂ **teaspoon**	baking powder	2 milliliters

Cream together margarine, peanut butter and sugar replacements. Add egg, water and vanilla, beating until fluffy. Combine flour, baking soda and baking powder in sifter and sift dry ingredients into creamed mixture. Stir to blend completely. Chill thoroughly, at least 2 hours or overnight. Drop by teaspoonfuls onto lightly greased cookie sheets, 2 to 3 inches (5 to 7 centimeters) apart. Press flat with a floured bottom of a small glass. Bake at 375°F (190°C) for 12 to 15 minutes.

Yield: 42 cookies
Exchange: (1 cookie) ¹/₃ bread
Calories: (1 cookie) 34

CORNFLAKE COOKIES

2	egg whites	2
¹/₂ **teaspoon**	salt	2 milliliters
1 teaspoon	white vinegar	5 milliliters
1 teaspoon	vanilla extract	5 milliliters
2 teaspoons	granulated sugar replacement	10 milliliters
1 teaspoon	liquid fructose	5 milliliters
2¹/₂ cups	unsweetened cornflakes (crushed)	625 milliliters

Beat egg whites until frothy. Add salt and continue beating until stiff. Beat in vinegar, vanilla, sugar replacement and liquid fructose; lightly fold in cornflakes. Drop by teaspoonfuls onto greased cookie sheets, 2 to 3 inches (5 to 7 centimeters) apart. Bake at 350°F (175°C) for 12 to 15 minutes, or until lightly browned.

Yield: 42 cookies
Exchange: (3 cookies) ¹/₃ fruit
Calories: (3 cookies) 21

APPLESAUCE COOKIES

¹/₄ **cup**	margarine	60 milliliters
1 tablespoon	granulated sugar replacement	15 milliliters
¹/₂ **cup**	unsweetened applesauce	125 milliliters
2 tablespoons	water	30 milliliters
1 cup	flour	250 milliliters
¹/₂ **teaspoon**	baking soda	2 milliliters
¹/₂ **teaspoon**	cinnamon	2 milliliters
¹/₄ **teaspoon**	salt	1 milliliter
¹/₄ **teaspoon**	cloves (ground)	1 milliliter
¹/₄ **cup**	raisins (chopped)	60 milliliters

Cream together margarine and sugar replacement. Add applesauce and water, stirring to mix well. Combine flour, baking soda, cinnamon, salt and cloves in sifter. Sift dry ingredients into applesauce mixture; stir to blend. Fold in raisins. Drop by teaspoonfuls onto lightly greased cookie sheet. Bake at 375°F (190°C) for 10 to 12 minutes.

Microwave: Place 6 to 8 cookies on waxed paper. Cook on LOW for 3 to 4 minutes, or until tops are set.

Yield: 30 cookies
Exchange: (1 cookie) ¹/₂ fruit, ¹/₅ fat
Calories: (1 cookie) 33

CINNAMON COOKIES

2	eggs	2
2 tablespoons	water	30 milliliters
5 teaspoons	granulated sugar replacement	25 milliliters
1 teaspoon	cinnamon	5 milliliters
1¹/₂ cups	flour	375 milliliters
¹/₂ **teaspoon**	baking soda	2 milliliters
¹/₄ **teaspoon**	salt	1 milliliter

Beat eggs and water until light and fluffy. Beat in sugar replacement and cinnamon. Combine flour, baking soda and salt in sifter; sift half of the dry ingredients over egg mixture. Fold to completely blend. Repeat with remaining dry ingredients. Drop by teaspoonfuls onto greased cookie sheet, 2 to 3 inches (5 to 7 centimeters) apart. Bake at 375°F (190°C) for 10 to 12 minutes.

Yield: 20 cookies
Exchange: (1 cookie) ¹/₂ bread
Calories: (1 cookie) 41

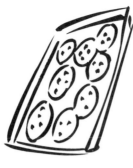

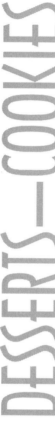

CHOCOLATE CHIP COOKIES

¼ cup	margarine	60 milliliters
1 tablespoon	granulated fructose	15 milliliters
1	egg	1
3 tablespoons	water	45 milliliters
1 teaspoon	vanilla extract	5 milliliters
¾ cup	flour	190 milliliters
¼ teaspoon	baking soda	1 milliliter
¼ teaspoon	salt	1 milliliter
½ cup	small semisweet chocolate chips	125 milliliters

Cream together margarine and fructose; beat in egg, water and vanilla extract. Combine flour, baking soda and salt in sifter. Sift dry ingredients into creamed mixture, stirring to blend thoroughly. Stir in chocolate chips. Drop by teaspoonfuls onto lightly greased cookie sheet, 2 inches (5 centimeters) apart. Bake at 375°F (190°C) for 8 to 10 minutes.

Yield: 30 cookies
Exchange: (1 cookie) ½ fruit, ½ fat
Calories: (1 cookie) 41

WALNUT KISSES

3	egg whites (beaten stiff)	3
2 tablespoons	granulated sugar replacement or granulated fructose	30 milliliters
2 tablespoons	cake flour (sifted)	30 milliliters
⅓ cup	walnuts (chopped fine)	90 milliliters
½ teaspoon	vanilla extract	2 milliliters

Beat sugar replacement into stiff egg whites. Sprinkle flour over egg white mixture; gently fold flour into egg whites with wire whisk or wooden spoon. Fold in walnuts and vanilla. Drop by teaspoonfuls onto lightly greased cookie sheets. Bake at 325°F (165°C) for 10 minutes. Remove from pan immediately.

Yield: 36 cookies
Exchange: (6 cookies with sugar replacement) ⅓ milk
Calories: (6 cookies with sugar replacement) 63

Exchange: (6 cookies with fructose) ½ milk
Calories: (6 cookies with fructose) 78

HERMIT COOKIES

¹/₂ cup	shortening	125 milliliters
3 tablespoons	granulated brown sugar replacement	45 milliliters
1	egg	1
1¹/₂ cups	flour (sifted)	375 milliliters
1 teaspoon	baking powder	5 milliliters
1 teaspoon	cinnamon	5 milliliters
¹/₄ teaspoon	salt	1 milliliter
¹/₄ teaspoon	baking soda	1 milliliter
¹/₄ teaspoon	nutmeg	1 milliliter
¹/₄ teaspoon	cloves (ground)	1 milliliter
¹/₃ cup	skim milk	90 milliliters
¹/₃ cup	raisins (chopped)	90 milliliters
¹/₄ cup	walnuts (chopped)	60 milliliters

Cream together shortening and brown sugar replacement. Add egg; beat until light and fluffy. Combine flour, baking powder, cinnamon, salt, baking soda, nutmeg and cloves in sifter; add alternately with milk to creamed mixture. Fold in raisins and walnuts. Drop by teaspoonfuls onto lightly greased baking sheets, 2 to 3 inches (5 to 7 centimeters) apart. Bake at 350°F (175°C) for 12 to 15 minutes.

> **Yield:** 48 cookies
> **Exchange:** (1 cookie) ¹/₃ fruit, ¹/₂ fat
> **Calories:** (1 cookie) 40

FATTEGMAND

2	eggs	2
1 tablespoon	granulated sugar replacement	15 milliliters
3 tablespoons	evaporated skimmed milk	45 milliliters
¹/₄ teaspoon	salt	1 milliliter
2 cups	flour	500 milliliters
	oil for deep-fat frying	

Combine all ingredients, except oil; mix just until blended. Roll out on lightly floured surface and form into 70 thin strips. Fry in deep fat, heated to 365°F (180°C), until golden brown. Remove to absorbent paper.

> **Yield:** 70 cookies
> **Exchange:** (2 cookies) ¹/₃ bread
> **Calories:** (2 cookies) 28

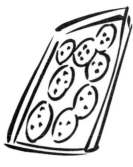

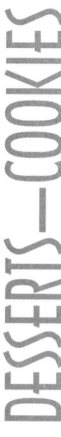

PUMPKIN BARS

1/3 cup	margarine	90 milliliters
1/4 cup	granulated brown sugar replacement	60 milliliters
1	egg	1
2 tablespoons	water	30 milliliters
1/2 cup	unsweetened pumpkin puree	125 milliliters
1 1/2 cups	flour	325 milliliters
1 teaspoon	allspice	5 milliliters

Cream margarine until fluffy. Add brown sugar replacement, egg and water, beating until completely blended. Beat in pumpkin puree, stir in flour and allspice, and mix to completely blend. Spread evenly in greased 13 x 9-inch (33 x 23-centimeter) cookie sheet. Bake at 350°F (175°C) for 16 to 18 minutes, or until sides pull away from pan. Cool and cut into bars.

> **Yield:** 48 cookies
> **Exchange:** (2 cookies) 1/3 bread, 1/2 fat
> **Calories:** (2 cookies) 52

FRUIT COOKIES

1/2 cup	margarine	125 milliliters
4 teaspoons	granulated sugar replacement	20 milliliters
2	eggs	2
2 cups	flour (sifted)	500 milliliters
1/2 teaspoon	baking soda	2 milliliters
1/4 teaspoon	salt	1 milliliter
1/2 teaspoon	nutmeg	2 milliliters
1/4 cup	hot apple juice	60 milliliters
1/4 cup	raisins (chopped)	60 milliliters
1/4 cup	currants	60 milliliters

Cream together margarine and sugar replacement. Add eggs; beat until fluffy. Combine flour, baking soda, salt and nutmeg in sifter; add alternately with hot apple juice to creamed mixture. Fold in raisins and currants. Allow to rest 15 minutes. Drop by teaspoonfuls onto lightly greased cookie sheet, 2 to 3 inches (5 to 7 centimeters) apart. Bake at 350°F (175°C) for 12 to 15 minutes.

> **Yield:** 60 cookies
> **Exchange:** (1 cookie) 1/2 fruit
> **Calories:** (1 cookie) 27

BANANA COOKIES

¹/₄ **cup**	margarine (soft)	60 milliliters
1 medium	banana	1 medium
1 teaspoon	vanilla extract	5 milliliters
1	egg	1
1 tablespoon	liquid fructose	15 milliliters
1 teaspoon	baking powder	5 milliliters
dash	salt	dash
1¹/₂ **cups**	flour	375 milliliters

Combine margarine, banana, vanilla, egg and fructose in mixing bowl. Beat until smooth. Add baking powder, salt and flour, mixing to blend well. Drop by teaspoonfuls onto lightly greased cookie sheets. Bake at 375°F (190°C) for 8 to 10 minutes.

Yield: 40 cookies
Exchange: (1 cookie) ¹/₂ fruit, ¹/₃ fat
Calories: (1 cookie) 32

CARROT COOKIES

¹/₂ **cup**	margarine	125 milliliters
1 tablespoon	granulated brown sugar replacement	15 milliliters
2 teaspoons	granulated sugar replacement	10 milliliters
1	egg	1
2 tablespoons	water	30 milliliters
1 teaspoon	vanilla extract	5 milliliters
1 cup	cooked carrots (mashed)	250 milliliters
2 cups	flour	500 milliliters
¹/₂ **teaspoon**	salt	2 milliliters
2 teaspoons	baking powder	10 milliliters

Cream together margarine and sugar replacements. Add egg, water and vanilla, beating until light and fluffy, and beat in carrots. Combine flour, salt and baking powder in sifter. Sift dry ingredients into carrot mixture; stir to blend completely. Drop by teaspoonfuls onto lightly greased cookie sheets. Bake at 375°F (190°C) for 10 to 12 minutes.

Microwave: Place 6 to 8 cookies on waxed paper. Cook on LOW for 3 to 4 minutes, or until tops are set.

Yield: 50 cookies
Exchange: (1 cookie) ¹/₂ vegetable
Calories: (1 cookie) 35

DESSERTS—COOKIES

PINEAPPLE DROPS

1/4 cup	margarine	60 milliliters
1 tablespoon	granulated brown sugar replacement	15 milliliters
1 tablespoon	granulated sugar replacement	15 milliliters
1	egg	1
1 teaspoon	pineapple flavoring	5 milliliters
1 1/4 cups	flour (sifted)	310 milliliters
1/2 teaspoon	baking powder	2 milliliters
1/4 teaspoon	baking soda	1 milliliter
1/2 cup	unsweetened crushed pineapple (with juice)	125 milliliters

Cream together margarine and sugar replacements. Add egg and pineapple flavoring, beating until fluffy. Combine flour, baking powder and baking soda in sifter. Add alternately with crushed pineapple (and juice) to creamed mixture, mixing thoroughly. Drop by teaspoonfuls onto lightly greased cookie sheets, 2 to 3 inches (5 to 7 centimeters) apart. Bake at 375°F (190°C) for 10 to 12 minutes.

Yield: 36 cookies
Exchange: (1 cookie) 1/3 fruit
Calories: (1 cookie) 29

BROWNIES

1/2 teaspoon	baking powder	2 milliliters
1/2 teaspoon	salt	2 milliliters
3 ounces	unsweetened chocolate (melted)	90 grams
1/2 cup	shortening (soft)	125 milliliters
2	eggs (beaten)	2
2 tablespoons	granulated sugar replacement	30 milliliters
1 1/2 cups	flour	375 milliliters
1 teaspoon	vanilla extract	5 milliliters

Combine all ingredients and beat vigorously until well blended. Spread mixture into greased 8-inch (20-centimeter)-square pan. Bake at 350°F (175°C) for 30 to 35 minutes. Cut into 2-inch (5-centimeter) squares.

Microwave: Cook on MEDIUM for 8 to 10 minutes, or until puffed and dry on top. Cut into 2-inch (5-centimeter) squares.

Yield: 16 cookies
Exchange: (1 brownie) 1 1/2 bread, 1 1/2 fat
Calories: (1 brownie) 136

TOFFEE SQUARES

¹/₂ **cup**	margarine	125 milliliters
3 tablespoons	granulated sugar replacement	45 milliliters
2	eggs	2
2 tablespoons	water	30 milliliters
2 cups	flour	500 milliliters
1 teaspoon	cinnamon	5 milliliters
1	egg white (slightly beaten)	1
¹/₂ **cup**	pecans (chopped fine)	125 milliliters

Cream margarine and sugar replacement until fluffy. Beat in whole eggs, one at a time. Add water, flour and cinnamon, mixing thoroughly. Spread into well-greased 15 x 10-inch (39 x 25-centimeter) cookie sheet. Pat with hand to level the surface. Brush beaten egg white over entire surface, and sprinkle evenly with chopped pecans. Slightly press pecans into cookie dough. Bake at 300°F (150°C) for about 40 to 45 minutes, or until done. Cut into 1¹/₂-inch (3³/₄-centimeter) squares.

Yield: 72 cookies
Exchange: (2 cookies) ¹/₃ bread, 1 fat
Calories: (2 cookies) 60

CHOCOLATE TEA COOKIES

¹/₄ **cup**	shortening (soft)	60 milliliters
3 tablespoons	granulated sugar replacement	45 milliliters
1	egg	1
¹/₂ **teaspoon**	vanilla extract	2 milliliters
2 tablespoons	skim milk	30 milliliters
1¹/₄ cups	cake flour (sifted)	310 milliliters
1-ounce square	unsweetened baking chocolate (melted)	28-gram square

Cream shortening. Add sugar replacement, egg, vanilla and milk, blending well. Add half the sifted flour; mix to completely blend. Stir in melted chocolate and remaining flour. With cookie press, press onto ungreased cookie sheets. Bake at 350°F (175°C) for 20 to 22 minutes.

Yield: 36 cookies
Exchange: (1 cookie) ¹/₅ bread; ¹/₃ fat
Calories: (1 cookie) 32

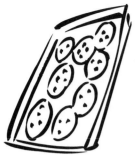

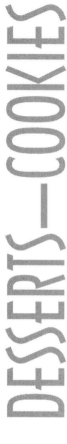

SPICED PRESSED COOKIES

$^1/_3$ cup	shortening (soft)	90 milliliters
3 tablespoons	granulated sugar replacement	45 milliliters
$1^1/_2$ teaspoons	vanilla extract	7 milliliters
3 tablespoons	water	45 milliliters
3	eggs	3
$2^1/_2$ cups	cake flour	625 milliliters
3 teaspoons	baking powder	15 milliliters
2 teaspoons	cinnamon	10 milliliters
1 teaspoon	nutmeg	5 milliliters
$^1/_2$ teaspoon	clove (ground)	2 milliliters

Combine shortening and sugar replacement in mixing bowl; beat until light and fluffy. Combine vanilla extract, water and eggs in measuring cup, beating until blended. Combine cake flour, baking powder and spices in sifter. Sift flour mixture alternately with egg mixture into shortening. Blend well after each addition. Chill thoroughly (at least 2 hours). With cookie press, press into shapes on ungreased cookie sheet. Bake at 425°F (220°C) for 7 to 8 minutes. Remove from pan immediately.

Yield: 60 cookies
Exchange: (1 cookie) $^1/_5$ bread, $^1/_3$ fat
Calories: (1 cookie) 27

CHINESE CHEWS

$^3/_4$ cup	cake flour	190 milliliters
$^3/_4$ teaspoon	baking powder	4 milliliters
3 tablespoons	granulated sugar replacement	45 milliliters
$^1/_8$ teaspoon	salt	$^1/_2$ milliliter
1 cup	dates (finely chopped)	250 milliliters
1 cup	walnuts (finely chopped)	250 milliliters
$^1/_4$ cup	water	60 milliliters

Sift together cake flour, baking powder, sugar replacement, and salt. Add dates and walnuts. Slowly add water and stir to make a soft dough. Spread in well-greased 8-inch (20-centimeter) square pan. Bake at 350°F (175°C) for about 40 minutes. Score into 1-inch ($2^1/_2$-centimeter) squares while warm.

Yield: 64 cookies
Exchange: (1 cookie) $^1/_3$ bread
Calories: (1 cookie) 24

CHOCOLATE-COCONUT DROPS

1/3 cup	margarine	90 milliliters
2 tablespoons	granulated brown sugar replacement	30 milliliters
1 teaspoon	vanilla extract	5 milliliters
2	eggs	2
1 1/2 cups	flour	375 milliliters
1/2 cup	cocoa	125 milliliters
1/2 teaspoon	salt	2 milliliters
1 teaspoon	baking soda	5 milliliters
1/3 cup	skim milk	90 milliliters
1/2 cup	unsweetened coconut (grated)	125 milliliters

Cream together margarine and brown sugar replacement. Beat in vanilla and eggs until light and fluffy. Sift flour, cocoa, salt and baking soda together; add alternately with milk to creamed mixture. Stir until well blended. Fold in coconut. Drop by teaspoonfuls onto lightly greased cookie sheets. Bake at 375°F (190°C) for 10 to 12 minutes.

Microwave: Place 6 to 8 cookies on waxed paper. Cook on LOW for 3 to 4 minutes, or until tops are set. Cool.

Yield: 40 cookies
Exchange: (1 cookie) 1/5 bread, 1/2 fat
Calories: (1 cookie) 39

PEANUT-BUTTER BALLS

1 cup	margarine (soft)	250 milliliters
2 tablespoons	granulated sugar replacement	30 milliliters
1 teaspoon	vanilla extract	5 milliliters
2 tablespoons	water	30 milliliters
2 cups	flour	500 milliliters
1	egg white (beaten)	1
1/2 cup	peanuts (very finely chopped)	125 milliliters

Beat margarine with sugar replacement until creamy. Add vanilla extract, water and flour, mixing well. Refrigerate 1 hour. Form into 1-inch (2 1/2-centimeter) balls, dip into beaten egg white and roll in chopped peanuts. Place on ungreased cookie sheets. Bake at 350°F (175°C) for 10 to 12 minutes.

Yield: 54 cookies
Exchange: (1 cookie) 1/3 fruit, 1 fat
Calories: (1 cookie) 56

DESSERTS—COOKIES

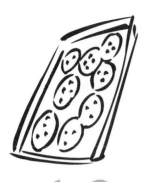

DREAM BARS

¹/₃ **cup**	margarine (soft)	90 milliliters
¹/₄ **cup**	granulated brown sugar replacement	60 milliliters
1 cup	flour	250 milliliters

Crust: Combine all ingredients in pastry blender or food processor until crumbly. Pat into 13 x 19-inch (33 x 23-centimeter) cookie pan. Bake at 375°F (190°C) for 10 minutes. Remove and cool.

2	eggs	2
¹/₄ **cup**	granulated brown sugar replacement	60 milliliters
2 tablespoons	flour	30 milliliters
1 teaspoon	baking powder	5 milliliters
¹/₄ **teaspoon**	salt	1 milliliter
1 teaspoon	vanilla extract	5 milliliters
1 tablespoon	water	15 milliliters
²/₃ **cup**	unsweetened coconut (grated)	190 milliliters
¹/₂ **cup**	walnuts (chopped fine)	125 milliliters

Topping: Beat eggs and stir in remaining ingredients until well blended. Pour over baked crust, spreading evenly. Bake at 375°F (190°C) for 20 minutes, or until set. Cool slightly. Cut into 48 bars with a sharp knife.

Yield: 48 cookies
Exchange: (1 cookie) ¹/₅ bread, ¹/₅ fat
Calories: (1 cookie) 37

CHOCOLATE WAFERS

¹/₄ **cup**	margarine (soft)	60 milliliters
4 teaspoons	granulated sugar replacement	20 milliliters
1	egg	1
2 tablespoons	cocoa	30 milliliters
1 teaspoon	vanilla extract	5 milliliters
1 cup	flour	250 milliliters
1 teaspoon	baking powder	5 milliliters
¹/₄ **teaspoon**	baking soda	1 milliliter
dash	salt	dash
2 tablespoons	water	30 milliliters

Combine margarine, sugar replacement, egg, cocoa and vanilla in mixing bowl or food processor. With electric mixer or steel blade, whip until creamy. Add flour, baking powder, baking soda, salt and water; mix well. Shape into balls. Wrap in waxed paper or plastic wrap. Chill at least 1 hour or overnight. Roll out dough to ⅛-inch (3-milliliter) thickness on lightly floured surface. Cut with 2½-inch (6¼-centimeter) round cookie cutter and place on ungreased cookie sheets. Bake at 350°F (175°C) for 8 to 10 minutes.

Yield: 30 wafers
Exchange: (1 wafer) ⅓ vegetable
Calories: (1 wafer) 29

CHRISTMAS CUTOUTS

½ cup	shortening (soft)	125 milliliters
3 tablespoons	granulated sugar replacement	45 milliliters
1	egg	1
2½ cups	cake flour	625 milliliters
2 teaspoons	baking powder	10 milliliters
½ teaspoon	salt	2 milliliters
½ cup	skim milk	125 milliliters
2 tablespoons	water	30 milliliters
1 teaspoon	vanilla extract	5 milliliters

Cream shortening. Add sugar replacement and egg; beat well. Combine cake flour, baking powder and salt in sifter. Combine milk, water and vanilla in measuring cup. Sift flour mixture alternately with milk into creamed mixture, mixing well after each addition. Chill thoroughly. Roll out to ¹⁄₁₆-inch (1.5-millimeter) thickness on pastry cloth, cut with cookie cutter, and decorate. Bake at 375-400°F (190-200°C) for 6 to 10 minutes.

Yield: 100 2-inch (5-centimeter) cookies
Exchange: (3 cookies) ⅓ bread
Calories: (3 cookies) 58

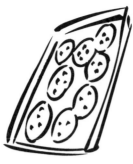

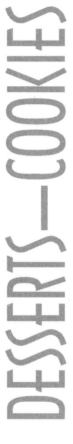

WALNUT PARTY COOKIES

¹/₂ **cup**	margarine (soft)	125 milliliters
2 tablespoons	granulated sugar replacement	30 milliliters
dash	salt	dash
1 teaspoon	vanilla extract	5 milliliters
1¹/₂ cups	cake flour (sifted)	375 milliliters
24	walnut halves	24

Combine margarine, sugar replacement, salt and vanilla in medium mixing bowl. Beat until light and fluffy. Stir in cake flour and refrigerate dough for at least 1 hour. Form dough into 24 small balls, place on ungreased cookie sheet and press walnut half into top of each cookie ball. Bake at 350°F (175°C) for 20 minutes, or until done.

Microwave: Place 6 to 8 cookie balls in circle on waxed paper; press walnut half into top of each. Cook on LOW for 5 to 6 minutes.

Yield: 24 cookies
Exchange: (1 cookie) ¹/₂ fruit, 1 fat
Calories: (1 cookie) 55

DESSERTS FOR SPECIAL OCCASIONS

In this section we present desserts that take a little more effort but that are spectacular. None requires special skill, however. In the case of soufflés, the only tricky part is that they need to be served shortly after they come out of the oven.

Many people enjoy serving special desserts at parties or when the whole family gathers together. With some of the recipes in this section, we suggest you get people to join in on the fun of assembling. For example, you might have an evening get-together where people assemble their own napoleons.

GRAND MARNIER SOUFFLÉ for Six

2 tablespoons	margarine or butter	30 milliliters
2¹/₂ tablespoons	regular all-purpose flour	37 milliliters
³/₄ cup	skim milk	190 milliliters
1 packet	concentrated acesulfame-K	1 packet
2	egg yolks (beaten)	2
3	egg whites	3
¹/₈ teaspoon	cream of tartar	¹/₂ milliliter
3 tablespoons	Grand Marnier	45 milliliters

The tricky part of souffles is to serve them right away when they are all puffed up.

In a saucepan melt the margarine or butter and remove it from the heat. Stir in the flour and milk; cook, stirring over medium heat, until thickened and smooth. Stir in the acesulfame-K; cool slightly; add egg yolks.

In a medium bowl, beat the egg whites until foamy; add the cream of tartar, beating until stiff peaks form when the beater is raised. Gently fold the egg yolk mixture and Grand Marnier into the egg whites. Turn into a one-quart soufflé dish or casserole coated with non-stick cooking spray.

Bake for 10 minutes in a preheated 450°F (230°C) oven, then turn down the heat to 325°F (165°C) and bake 15 minutes longer. Serve immediately.

Yield:	6 servings	
Exchange:	1 fat, 1 bread	
Each serving:	Calories: 122	Fiber: trace
	Sodium: 27 milligrams	Cholesterol: 34 milligrams

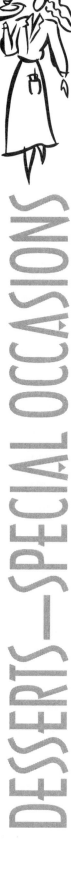

GRAND MARNIER SOUFFLÉ for Eight

1¹/₂ **cups**	nonfat milk	375 milliliters
2 **tablespoons**	margarine or butter	30 milliliters
3 **tablespoons**	flour	45 milliliters
¹/₄ **cup**	egg substitute	60 milliliters
2 **tablespoons**	fructose	30 milliliters
¹/₃ **cup**	measures-like-sugar saccharin	90 milliliters
7 **packets**	acesulfame-K	7 packets
2 **teaspoons**	vanilla extract	10 milliliters
1¹/₂ **teaspoons**	orange extract	7 milliliters
3 **tablespoons**	orange-flavored liqueur such as Grand Marnier (optional)	45 milliliters
4	egg whites	4
¹/₂ **teaspoon**	cream of tartar	2 milliliters
2 **tablespoons**	measures-like-sugar aspartame	30 milliliters

Grand Marnier is a special liqueur. Those who prefer to avoid alcohol, even when it cooks out, can make this souffle without it. Those who want to try the Grand Marnier may want to buy a very small ("nip") bottle, as the liqueur is expensive.

Heat the milk just to the boiling point and set it aside. In a separate saucepan, melt the margarine over low heat and add flour. Stir together for two minutes over low-to-medium heat, stirring constantly. Turn off the heat. Whisk in the hot milk, stirring constantly. Cook over medium heat, until the mixture thickens. Turn off the heat. Slowly stir in the egg substitute. Then stir in the fructose, saccharin, acesulfame-K, vanilla and orange extracts, and liqueur, if using. Set aside.

In a separate bowl, beat the egg whites and cream of tartar and continue beating until stiff. Mix a small amount of the beaten egg whites into the milk mixture to lighten it. Then use a rubber spatula to fold in the rest of the beaten egg whites. Pour the mixture into a souffle dish that has been coated with non-stick cooking spray. Bake in a preheated 375° F (190°C) oven for 20 minutes. Do not overbake. As soon as the souffle is out of the oven, use a small sieve to dust aspartame over the top.

Yield:	8 servings	
Exchange:	¹/₂ fruit, ¹/₂ meat	
Each serving:	Calories: 78	Fiber: trace
	Sodium: 97 milligrams	Cholesterol: trace

CHOCOLATE SOUFFLÉ

½ cup	unsweetened cocoa powder	125 milliliters
2 tablespoons	powdered sugar	30 milliliters
½ cup	measures-like-sugar saccharin	125 milliliters
7 packets	concentrated acesulfame-K	7 packets
2 tablespoons	cornstarch	30 milliliters
dash	salt (optional)	dash
½ cup	nonfat milk	125 milliliters
½ cup	water	125 milliliters
4	egg whites	4
½ teaspoon	cream of tartar	2 milliliters
¼ cup	egg substitute	60 milliliters
1 teaspoon	vanilla extract	5 milliliters
2 tablespoons	measures-like-sugar aspartame	30 milliliters

This is absolutely wonderful.

Sift the cocoa, sugar, saccharin and acesulfame-K, salt, and cornstarch together twice. Put them in the top of a double boiler and add the nonfat milk and water. Whisk constantly while cooking until the mixture is smooth and thick, about eight minutes. Remove from the heat. Beat the egg whites with an electric mixer until they hold their shape; add the cream of tartar, and continue beating until stiff peaks form. Pour the egg substitute and vanilla extract into the chocolate mixture. Mix. Add a small amount of the beaten egg whites into the chocolate mixture to lighten. Then use a rubber spatula to fold in the rest of the egg whites.

Pour into a 6-cup (1.5-liter) soufflé dish that has been coated with non-stick cooking spray. Bake in a preheated 400°F (200°C) oven for 20 minutes. Do not overcook; the center will be a little runny to make a sauce. As soon as the soufflé is out of the oven, dust aspartame over the top.

Yield:	8 servings	
Exchange:	½ bread	
Each serving:	Calories: 54	Fiber: 0
	Sodium: 84 milligrams	Cholesterol: trace

DESSERTS—SPECIAL OCCASIONS

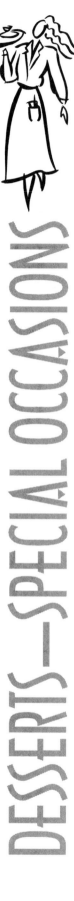

HOT APPLE SOUFFLÉ

1/2 cup	margarine or butter	125 milliliters
1/2 cup	flour	125 milliliters
2 cups	cold skim milk	500 milliliters
2 tablespoons	granulated sugar	30 milliliters
1 packet	concentrated acesulfame-K	1 packet
2	medium apples	2
4	eggs (separated)	4
2 tablespoons	toasted almonds (slivered)	30 milliliters
	grated peel from 1/2 lemon	

This makes the house smell wonderful when it's baking and tastes great, too.

About 2¼ hours before serving, melt the margarine in a medium saucepan; stir in the flour, then the milk. Cook, stirring constantly, until smooth and thickened. Blend in the sugar, acesulfame-K, and lemon peel; let cool slightly, stirring occasionally.

Meanwhile, wash, pare, and core the apples, then cut each into about 10 lengthwise wedges. Arrange them evenly over the bottom of a casserole which measures 8 cups (2 liters) to the brim. Beat the egg whites until stiff. Blend the yolks into the flour-milk mixture, then carefully fold in the egg whites. Pour this mixture over the apples, then sprinkle it with almonds. Bake in a preheated 325°F (165°C) oven for 1¼ hours or until light brown and firm. Serve at once.

Yield:	8 servings		
Exchange:	1 bread, 1/2 meat, 1 fat		
Each serving:	Calories: 229	Fiber: 1 gram	
	Sodium: 67 milligrams	Cholesterol: 138 milligrams	

BERRY SOUFFLÉ

1³/₄ cups	mixed red berries (fresh or frozen—unsweetened, thawed & drained)	440 milliliters
1 tablespoon	Chambord or fruit-flavored liqueur (optional) or—	15 milliliters
2 teaspoons	strawberry extract	10 milliliters
5	egg whites	5

A lovely and impressive soufflé that tastes as good as it looks.

In a blender or food processor, puree the berries and liqueur. In a mixing bowl, beat the egg whites until stiff but not dry. Fold the puree into the egg whites. Spoon the mixture into a two-quart soufflé dish coated with non-stick cooking spray. Place the soufflé dish on a cooking sheet and bake for 30 to 35 minutes at 350°F (175°C). Serve immediately.

Yield:	6 servings	
Exchange:	½ milk	
Each serving:	Calories: 31	Fiber: 2 grams
	Sodium: 42 milligrams	Cholesterol: 0

CRÊPES

1 packet	concentrated acesulfame-K	1 packet
1 cup	skim milk	250 milliliters
2 tablespoons	safflower oil	30 milliliters
½ cup	egg substitute	125 milliliters
½ cup	flour	125 milliliters
2 teaspoons	baking powder	10 milliliters
¼ teaspoon	vanilla extract	1 milliliter

This recipe makes 14 five-inch (13-centimeter) crêpes. You can make them in a larger skillet and use strawberry or blueberry topping or a different fruit filling such as fruit-only jam.

Combine all the ingredients in a blender and blend for a minute or so or mix in an electric mixer until the batter is smooth. Heat a small, oiled skillet or crêpe pan until a drop of water "dances" when you splash it on the hot surface. Add ⅓ cup (90 milliliters) of the batter and move the pan around so the batter covers evenly. Cook over medium heat on one side until the edges are browned and there are bubbles throughout the crêpe. Turn and cook on the other side to brown. Spoon 1 tablespoon (15 milliliters) of strawberry topping on each crêpe and roll the crêpes up. Top with a dollop of your favorite whipped topping.

Yield:	14 crêpes	
Exchange:	½ fat	
Each serving:	Calories: 44	Fiber: trace
	Sodium: 28 milligrams	Cholesterol: trace

TRADITIONAL CRÊPE FILLING

Nonfat ricotta cheese makes a nice crêpe filling, especially when flavored with a little nutmeg. Add aspartame if you want it sweeter. Adding a couple of sliced strawberries or raspberries is a nice touch. A whipped topping can also be used.

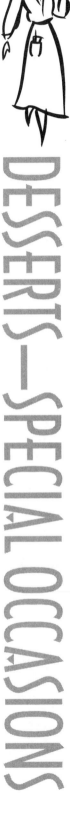

DESSERTS—SPECIAL OCCASIONS

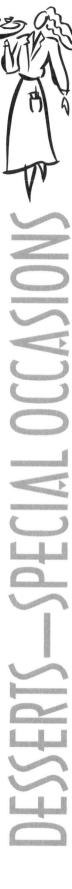

CRÊPES SUZETTES SAUCE

³/₄ **cup**	orange juice	190 milliliters
1 teaspoon	grated orange peel	5 milliliters
1¹/₂ teaspoons	cornstarch	7 milliliters
1 packet	concentrated acesulfame-K	1 packet
1 teaspoon	margarine or butter	5 milliliters
1 teaspoon	concentrated aspartame	5 milliliters
¹/₂ teaspoon	orange extract	2 milliliters
2 tablespoons	orange-flavored liqueur, such as Grand Marnier (optional)	30 milliliters

Crêpes suzettes are wonderful! We offer here a version that is much lower in fat and sweeteners. If you prefer to avoid liqueurs, double the amount of orange extract. You can serve this sauce over your choice of crêpes. Be sure to add together the calories and other values for both the sauce and the crêpe.

In a saucepan whisk together the orange juice, orange peel, cornstarch, and acesulfame-K. Heat to boiling, then immediately reduce the heat and cook over a medium flame, stirring constantly. When the mixture is thickened, turn off the heat.

Stir in the margarine, aspartame, orange extract, and liqueur if desired. Take each crêpe and fold in half, then again, and arrange on a separate plate. Spoon a little crêpes suzettes sauce over each.

Yield:	6 servings
Exchange:	free
Each serving:	Calories: 22
	Sodium: 7 milligrams

Fiber: trace
Cholesterol: 0

NO-FAT CRÊPES

1 cup	nonfat milk	250 milliliters
¹/₄ **cup**	egg substitute	60 milliliters
³/₄ **cup**	flour	190 milliliters
2 packets	acesulfame-K	2 packets
¹/₂ teaspoon	cinnamon	2 milliliters
1 teaspoon	sugar	5 milliliters

These crêpes work very well despite the lack of fat. They are easy to cook and easy to roll around fillings. The easiest crêpe fillings are a little nonfat ricotta cheese sweetened with aspartame and nutmeg or flavored applesauce.

Combine all the ingredients in a blender or food processor until smooth. Heat a non-stick omelette pan over medium-high heat. Spoon 2 tablespoons (30 milliliters) batter into the hot pan and roll the pan from side to side to cover the entire surface. When the edges curl away from the sides of the pan, turn the crêpe over. Repeat until all the batter is used. Store crêpes in a covered container with a piece of plastic wrap, waxed paper, or aluminum foil between each crêpe.

Yield: 12 crêpes
Exchange: ½ milk
Each serving: Calories: 38   Fiber: trace
Sodium: 22 milligrams   Cholesterol: trace

CHEESE FLAN

4	eggs or equivalent egg substitute	4
½ cup	nonfat sour cream	125 milliliters
8 ounces	nonfat cream cheese	250 grams
¼ cup	lemon juice	60 milliliters
2 teaspoons	vanilla extract	10 milliliters
1 packet	concentrated acesulfame-K	1 packet
dash	nutmeg	dash
4 tablespoons	chopped walnuts	60 milliliters
2 tablespoons	measures-like-sugar aspartame	30 milliliters
1	unbaked crust (optional)	1

You'll love serving this elegant dessert. It rivals the desserts in fancy restaurants, yet it's easy to make and virtually foolproof.

Put the first seven ingredients into a blender. Pour the blender contents onto a graham cracker or other crust, if desired. Bake at 375°F (190°C) for 25 minutes. Mix together the walnuts and aspartame. Sprinkle over the flan. Cool. Store the flan in the refrigerator.

Yield: 16 servings
Exchange: ½ milk
Each serving: Calories: 41   Fiber: trace
Sodium: 111 milligrams   Cholesterol: 3 milligrams

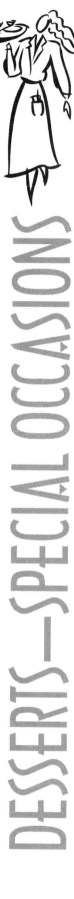

MOUSSE AU CHOCOLAT

2 teaspoons	unflavored gelatin	10 milliliters
¹/₄ cup	cold water	60 milliliters
¹/₃ cup	unsweetened cocoa powder	90 milliliters
1 teaspoon	cornstarch	5 milliliters
15 packets	concentrated acesulfame-K	15 packets
1 teaspoon	vanilla extract	5 milliliters
¹/₄ cup	skim milk	60 milliliters
1 packet	concentrated acesulfame-K	1 packet
1 (2¹/₂-ounce)	milk chocolate bar (made without chocolate)	1 (71-gram)
6 tablespoons	nonfat cream cheese	90 milliliters
4	egg whites	4
¹/₄ teaspoon	cream of tartar	1 milliliter

This is a genuinely rich mousse. Very creamy and satisfying. We used a "diabetic" candy bar with sorbitol.

Sprinkle the gelatin over the cold water to soften. In a saucepan, whisk together the cocoa, cornstarch, acesulfame-K, vanilla extract, and milk. Cook over medium heat for a few minutes, stirring with a wire whisk. Remove from the heat. Use a food processor or blender to chop the chocolate bar into small pieces; stir the chocolate into the cocoa mixture until smooth. Stir in the softened gelatin. Heat the cream cheese over low heat or in the microwave oven until softened. Add small amounts of the chocolate mixture to the softened cream cheese. Whisk until it is smooth and creamy and no small lumps remain. Use a rubber spatula to add this cream cheese–chocolate mixture back into the saucepan and whisk well to combine with the remaining chocolate.

Set the saucepan into a large bowl chilled with ice cubes and ice water to cool and thicken. In a separate bowl beat the egg whites until foamy; add the cream of tartar and continue beating until stiff peaks form. Put a small amount of the chocolate mixture into the beaten egg whites to lighten. Then use a rubber spatula to fold the rest of the egg whites into the chocolate mixture. Pour into eight small (¹/₂-cup or 125-milliliter) serving dishes and refrigerate until set.

Yield:	8 servings	
Exchange:	¹/₂ milk, ¹/₂ fat	
Each serving:	Calories: 81	Fiber: 0
	Sodium: 147 milligrams	Cholesterol: 3 milligrams

Foods are listed with their serving sizes, which are usually measured after cooking. When you begin, you should measure the size of each serving. This may help you learn to "eyeball" correct serving sizes.

The following chart shows the amount of nutrients in one serving from each list.

GROUPS/LISTS	Carbohydrate (grams)	Protein (grams)	Fat (grams)	Calories
Carbohydrate Group				
Starch	15	3	1 or less	80
Fruit	15	—	—	60
Milk				
Skim	12	8	0–3	90
Low-fat	12	8	5	120
Whole	12	8	8	150
Other carbohydrates	15	varies	varies	varies
Vegetables	5	2	—	25
Meat & Meat Substitute Group				
Very lean	—	7	0–1	35
Lean	—	7	3	55
Medium-fat	—	7	5	75
High-fat	—	7	8	100
Fat Group	—	—	5	45

The exchange list provides you with a lot of food choices (foods from the basic food groups, foods with added sugars, free foods, combination foods, and fast foods). This give you variety in your meals. Several foods, such as beans, peas, and lentils, bacon, and peanut butter, are on two lists. This gives you flexibility in putting your meals together. Whenever you choose new foods or vary your meal plan, monitor your blood glucose to see how these different foods affect your blood glucose level.

Most foods in the Carbohydrate group have about the same amount of carbohydrate per serving. You can exchange starch, fruit, or milk choices in your meal plan. Vegetables are in this group but contain only about 5 grams of carbohydrate.

A Word About Food Labels

Exchange information is based on foods found in grocery stores. However, food companies often change the ingredients in their products. This is why you need to check the Nutrition Facts panel of the food label.

The Nutrition Facts tell you the number of calories and grams of carbohydrate, protein, and fat in one serving. Compare these numbers with the exchange information in this book to see how many exchanges you will be eating. In this way, food labels can help you add foods to your meal plans.

Ask your dietitian to help you use food label information to plan your meals.

Getting Started!

See your dietician regularly when you are first learning how to use your meal plan and the exchange lists. Your meal plan can be adjusted to fit changes in your lifestyle, such as work, school, vacation, or travel. Regular nutrition counseling can help you make positive changes in your eating habits.

Careful eating habits will help you feel better and be healthier, too. Best wishes and good eating with *Exchange Lists for Meal Planning*.

EXCHANGE LISTS *(vertical, left margin)*

STARCH LIST

Cereals, grains, pasta, breads, crackers, snacks, starchy vegetables, and cooked beans, peas, and lentils are starches. In general, one starch is:

- $\frac{1}{2}$ cup of cereal, grain, pasta, or starchy vegetable,
- 1 ounce of a bread product, such as 1 slice of bread,
- $\frac{3}{4}$ to 1 ounce of most snack foods. (Some snack foods may also have added fat.)

Nutrition Tips
1. Most starch choices are good sources of B vitamins.
2. Foods made from whole grains are good sources of fiber.
3. Beans, peas, and lentils are a good source of protein and fiber.

Selection Tips
1. Choose starches made with little fat as often as you can.
2. Starchy vegetables prepared with fat count as one starch and one fat.
3. Bagels or muffins can be 2,3, or 4 starch choices. Check the size you eat.
4. Beans, peas, and lentils are also found on the Meat and Meat Substitutes list.
5. Regular potato chips and tortilla chips are found on the Other Carbohydrates list.
6. Most of the serving sizes are measured after cooking.
7. Always check Nutrition Facts on the food label.

> **One starch exchange equals**
> 15 grams carbohydrate,
> 3 grams protein,
> 0 to1 grams fat, &
> 80 calories.

BREAD

Bagel	$\frac{1}{2}$ (1 ounce)
Bread (reduced-calorie)	2 slices ($1\frac{1}{2}$ ounce)
Bread (white, whole-wheat, pumpernickel, rye)	1 slice (1 ounce)
Bread sticks (crisp, 4 inch x $\frac{1}{2}$ inch)	2 ($\frac{2}{3}$ ounce)
English muffin	$\frac{1}{2}$
Hot dog or hamburger bun	$\frac{1}{2}$ (1 ounce)
Pita (6 inches across)	$\frac{1}{2}$
Raisin bread (unfrosted)	1 slice (1 ounce)
Roll (plain, small)	1 (1 ounce)
Tortilla, corn (6 inches across)	1
Tortilla, flour (7–8 inches across)	1
Waffle ($4\frac{1}{2}$ inches square, reduced-fat)	1

CEREALS & GRAINS

Bran cereals	$\frac{1}{2}$ cup
Bulgur	$\frac{1}{2}$ cup
Cereals	$\frac{1}{2}$ cup

Cereals (unsweetened, ready-to-eat)	$^3/_4$ cup
Cornmeal (dry)	3 tablespoons
Couscous	$^1/_3$ cup
Flour (dry)	3 tablespoons
Granola (low-fat)	$^1/_4$ cup
Grape-Nuts®	$^1/_4$ cup
Grits	$^1/_2$ cup
Kasha	$^1/_2$ cup
Millet	$^1/_4$ cup
Muesli	$^1/_4$ cup
Oats	$^1/_2$ cup
Pasta	$^1/_2$ cup
Puffed cereal	$1^1/_2$ cups
Rice milk	$^1/_2$ cup
Rice, white or brown	$^1/_3$ cup
Shredded Wheat®	$^1/_2$ cup
Sugar-frosted cereal	$^1/_2$ cup
Wheat germ	3 tablespoons

STARCHY VEGETABLES

Baked beans	$^1/_3$ cup
Corn	$^1/_2$ cup
Corn on cob (medium)	1 (5 ounces)
Mixed vegetables (with corn, peas, or pasta)	1 cup
Peas (green)	$^1/_2$ cup
Plantain	$^1/_2$ cup
Potato (baked or boiled)	1 small (3 ounces)
Potato (mashed)	$^1/_2$ cup
Squash (winter, acorn, butternut)	1 cup
Yam, sweet potato (plain)	$^1/_2$ cup

CRACKERS & SNACKS

Animal crackers	8
Graham crackers ($2^1/_2$ inches square)	3
Matzoh	$^3/_4$ ounce
Melba toast	4 slices
Oyster crackers	24
Popcorn (popped, no fat added or low-fat microwave)	3 cups
Pretzels	$^3/_4$ ounce
Rice cakes (4 inches across)	2
Saltine-type crackers	6
Snack chips, fat-free (tortilla, potato)	15–20 ($^3/_4$ ounce)
Whole-wheat crackers (no fat added)	2–5 ($^3/_4$ ounce)

BEANS, PEAS, & LENTILS
(Count as 1 starch exchange, plus 1 very lean meat exchange)

Beans & peas (garbanzo, pinto, kidney, white, split, black-eyed)	½ cup
Lentils	½ cup
Lima beans	⅔ cup
Miso♣	3 tablespoons

♣ = 400 or more sodium per exchange.

STARCHY FOODS PREPARED WITH FAT
(Count as 1 starch exchange, plus 1 fat exchange)

Biscuit (2½ inches across)	1
Chow mein noodles	½ cup
Corn bread, (2 inch cube)	1 (2 ounces)
Crackers (round butter type)	6
Croutons	1 cup
French-fried potatoes	16 to 25 (3 ounces)
Granola	¼ cup
Muffin (small)	1 (1½ ounce)
Pancake (4 inches across)	2
Popcorn (microwave)	3 cups
Sandwich crackers (cheese or peanut butter filling)	3
Stuffing, bread (prepared)	⅓ cup
Taco shell (6 inches across)	2
Waffle (4½ inches square)	1
Whole-wheat crackers (fat added)	4 to 6 (1 ounce)

Starches often swell in cooking, so a small amount of un-cooked starch will become a much larger amount of cooked food. The following table shows some of the changes.

Food (Starch Group)	Uncooked	Cooked
Oatmeal	3 Tablespoons	½ cup
Cream of Wheat	2 Tablespoons	½ cup
Grits	3 Tablespoons	½ cup
Rice	2 Tablespoons	⅓ cup
Spaghetti	¼ cup	½ cup
Noodles	⅓ cup	½ cup
Macaroni	¼ cup	½ cup
Dried beans	¼ cup	½ cup
Dried peas	¼ cup	½ cup
Lentils	3 Tablespoons	½ cup

FRUIT LIST

Fresh, frozen, canned, and dried fruits and fruit juices are on this list. In general, one fruit exchange is:
- 1 small to medium fresh fruit,
- $1/2$ cup of canned or fresh fruit or fruit juice,
- $1/4$ cup of dried fruit.

Nutrition Tips
1. Fresh, frozen, and dried fruits have about 2 grams of fiber per choice. Fruit juices contain very little fiber.
2. Citrus fruits, berries, and melons are good sources of Vitamin C.

Selection Tips
1. Count $1/2$ cup cranberries or rhubarb sweetened with sugar substitutes as free foods.
2. Read the Nutrition Facts on the food label. If one serving has more than 15 grams of carbohydrate, you will need to adjust the size of the serving you eat or drink.
3. Portion sizes for canned fruits are for the fruit and a small amount of juice.
4. Whole fruit is more filling than fruit juice and may be a better choice.
5. Food labels for fruits may contain the words "no sugar added" or "unsweetened." This means that no sucrose (table sugar) has been added.
6. Generally, fruit canned in extra light syrup has the same amount of carbohydrate per serving as the "no sugar added" or the juice pack. All canned fruits on the fruit list are based on one of these three types of pack.

> **One fruit exchange equals**
> 15 grams carbohydrate
> & 60 calories.
> (The weight includes
> skin, core, seeds, and rind.)

FRUIT

Apple (unpeeled, small)	1 (4 ounces)
Applesauce (unsweetened)	$1/2$ cup
Apples (dried)	4 rings
Apricots (fresh)	4 whole ($5^1/2$ ounces)
Apricots (dried)	8 halves
Apricots (canned)	$1/2$ cup
Banana (small)	1 (4 ounces)
Blackberries	$3/4$ cup
Blueberries	$3/4$ cup
Cantaloupe (small)	$1/3$ melon (11 ounces) or 1 cup cubes
Cherries (sweet, fresh)	12 (3 ounces)
Cherries (sweet, canned)	$1/2$ cup
Dates	3
Figs (fresh)	$1^1/2$ large or 2 medium ($3^1/2$ ounces)
Figs (dried)	$1^1/2$

Fruit cocktail	$^1/_2$ cup
Grapefruit (large)	(11 ounces)
Grapefruit sections (canned)	$^3/_4$ cup
Grapes (small)	17 (3 ounces)
Honeydew melon	1 slice (10 ounces) or 1 cup cubes
Kiwi	1 (3$^1/_2$ ounces)
Mandarin oranges (canned)	$^3/_4$ cup
Mango (small)	$^1/_2$ fruit (5$^1/_2$ ounces) or $^1/_2$ cup
Nectarine (small)	1 (5 ounces)
Orange (small)	1 (6$^1/_2$ ounces)
Papaya	$^1/_2$ fruit (8 ounces) or 1 cup cubes
Peach (medium, fresh)	1 (6 ounces)
Peaches (canned)	$^1/_2$ cup
Pear (large, fresh)	$^1/_2$ (4 ounces)
Pears (canned)	$^1/_2$ cup
Pineapple (fresh)	$^3/_4$ cup
Pineapple (canned)	$^1/_2$ cup
Plums (small)	2 (5 ounces)
Plums (canned)	$^1/_2$ cup
Prunes (dried)	3
Raisins	2 Tablespoons
Raspberries	1 cup
Strawberries	1$^1/_4$ cup whole berries
Tangerines (small)	2 (8 ounces)
Watermelon	1 slice (13$^1/_2$ ounces) or 1$^1/_4$ cup cubes

FRUIT JUICE

Apple juice/cider	$^1/_2$ cup
Cranberry juice cocktail	$^1/_3$ cup
Cranberry juice cocktail (reduced-calorie)	1 cup
Fruit juice blends (100% juice)	$^1/_3$ cup
Grape juice	$^1/_3$ cup
Grapefruit juice	$^1/_2$ cup
Orange juice	$^1/_2$ cup
Pineapple juice	$^1/_2$ cup
Prune juice	$^1/_3$ cup

MILK LIST

Different types of milk and milk products are on this list. Cheeses are on the Meat list and cream and other dairy fats are on the Fat list. Based on the amount of fat they contain, milks are divided into skim/very low-fat milk, low-fat milk, and whole milk. One choice of these includes:

240

EXCHANGE LISTS

	Carbohydrate (grams)	Protein (grams)	Fat (grams)	Calories
Skim/very low-fat milk	12	8	0 to 3	90
Low-fat milk	12	8	5	120
Whole Milk	12	8	8	150

Nutrition Tips

1. Milk and yogurt are good sources of calcium and protein. Check the food label.
2. The higher the fat content of milk and yogurt, the greater the amount of saturated fat and cholesterol. Choose lower-fat varieties.
3. For those who are lactose intolerant, look for lactose-reduced or lactose-free varieties of milk.

Selection Tips

1. One cup equals 8 fluid ounces or 1/2 pint.
2. Look for chocolate milk, frozen yogurt, and ice cream on the Other Carbohydrates list.
3. Nondairy creamers are on the Free Foods list.
4. Look for rice milk on the Starch list.
5. Look for soy milk on the Medium-fat Meat list.

One milk exchange equals
12 grams carbohydrate
& 8 grams protein.

SKIM & VERY LOW-FAT MILK
(0 to 3 grams fat per serving)

Skim milk	1 cup
1/2 % milk	1 cup
1% milk	1 cup
Nonfat or low-fat buttermilk	1 cup
Evaporated skim milk	1/2 cup
Nonfat dry milk	1/3 cup dry
Plain nonfat yogurt	3/4 cup
Nonfat or low-fat fruit-flavored yogurt (sweetened with aspartame or with a nonnutritive sweetener)	1 cup

LOW-FAT MILK
(5 grams fat per serving)

2% milk	1 cup
Plain low-fat yogurt	3/4 cup
Sweet acidophilus milk	1 cup

241

WHOLE MILK
(8 grams fat per serving)

Whole milk	1 cup
Evaporated whole milk	½ cup
Goat's milk	1 cup
Kefir	1 cup

OTHER CARBOHYDRATES LIST

You can substitute food choices from this list for a starch, fruit, or milk choice on your meal plan. Some choices will also count as one or more fat choices.

Nutrition Tips

1. These foods can be substituted in your meal plan, even though they contain added sugars or fat. However, they do not contain as many important vitamins and minerals as the choices on the Starch, Fruit, or Milk list.
2. When planning to include these foods in your meal, be sure to include foods from all the lists to eat a balanced meal.

Selection Tips

1. Because many of these foods are concentrated sources of carbohydrate and fat, the portion sizes are often very small.
2. Always check Nutrition Facts on the food label. It will be your most accurate source of information.
3. Many fat-free or reduced-fat products made with fat replacers contain carbohydrate. When eaten in large amounts, they may need to be counted. Talk with your dietician to determine how to count these in your meal plan.
4. Look for fat-free salad dressings in smaller amounts on the Free Foods list.

> **One Exchange equals**
> 15 grams carbohydrate,
> or 1 starch, or 1 fruit, or 1 milk.

Food & Serving Size	Exchanges Per Serving
Angel food cake (unfrosted) *¹/₁₂th cake*	2 carbohydrates
Brownie (small, unfrosted) *2 inch square*	1 carbohydrate, 1 fat
Cake (unfrosted) *2 inch square*	1 carbohydrate, 1 fat
Cake (frosted) *2 inch square*	2 carbohydrates, 1 fat
Cookie (fat-free) *2 small*	1 carbohydrate
Cookie or sandwich cookie (with creme filling) *2 small*	1 carbohydrate, 1 fat
Cranberry sauce (jellied) *¼ cup*	1½ carbohydrates
Cupcake (frosted) *1 small*	2 carbohydrates, 1 fat
Doughnut (plain cake) *1 medium (1½ ounces)*	1½ carbohydrates, 2 fats
Doughnut (glazed) *3¾ inches across (2 ounces)*	2 carbohydrates, 2 fats
Fruit juice bars (frozen, 100% juice) *1 bar (3 ounces)*	1 carbohydrate

Fruit snacks, chewy (pureed fruit concentrate) *1 roll (³/₄ ounce)*	1 carbohydrate
Fruit spreads (100% fruit) *1 Tablespoon*	1 carbohydrate
Gelatin (regular) *¹/₂ cup*	1 carbohydrate
Gingersnaps *(3)*	1 carbohydrate
Granola bar *(1 bar)*	1 carbohydrate, 1 fat
Granola bar (fat-free) *1 bar*	2 carbohydrates
Hummus *¹/₃ cup*	1 carbohydrate, 1 fat
Ice cream *(¹/₂ cup)*	1 carbohydrate, 2 fats
Ice cream (light) *¹/₂ cup*	1 carbohydrate, 1 fat
Ice cream (fat-free, no sugar added) *¹/₂ cup*	1 carbohydrate
Jam or jelly (regular) *1 Tablespoon*	1 carbohydrate
Milk (chocolate, whole) *1 cup*	2 carbohydrates, 1 fat
Pie (fruit, 2 crusts) *¹/₆ pie*	3 carbohydrates, 2 fats
Pie (pumpkin or custard) *¹/₈ pie*	1 carbohydrate, 2 fats
Potato chips, *12 to18 (1 ounce)*	1 carbohydrate, 2 fats
Pudding, regular (made with low-fat milk) *¹/₂ cup*	2 carbohydrates
Pudding, sugar-free (made with low-fat milk) *¹/₂ cup*	1 carbohydrate
Salad dressing (fat-free)♣ *¹/₄ cup*	1 carbohydrate
Sherbet (sorbet) *¹/₂ cup*	2 carbohydrates
Spaghetti or pasta sauce (canned)♣ *¹/₂ cup*	1 carbohydrate, 1 fat
Sweet roll or Danish, *1 (2¹/₂ ounces)*	2¹/₂ carbohydrates, 2 fats
Syrup (light) *2 Tablespoons*	1 carbohydrate
Syrup (regular) *1 Tablespoon*	1 carbohydrate
Syrup (regular) *¹/₄ cup*	4 carbohydrates
Tortilla chips, *6 to 12 (1ounce)*	1 carbohydrate, 2 fats
Vanilla wafers *(5)*	1 carbohydrate, 1 fat
Yogurt (frozen, low-fat, fat-free) *¹/₃ cup*	1 carbohydrate, 0 to 1 fat
Yogurt (frozen, fat-free, no sugar added) *¹/₂ cup*	1 carbohydrate
Yogurt (low-fat with fruit) *1 cup*	3 carbohydrates, 0 to 1 fat

♣ = 400 mg or more sodium per exchange.

VEGETABLE LIST

Vegetables that contain small amounts of carbohydrates and calories are on this list. Vegetables contain important nutrients. Try to eat at least 2 or 3 vegetable choices each day. In general, one vegetable exchange is:
- ¹/₂ cup of cooked vegetables or vegetable juice,
- 1 cup of raw vegetables.

If you eat 1 to 2 vegetable choices at a meal or snack, you do not have to count the calories or carbohydrates because they contain small amounts of these nutrients.

Nutrition Tips

1. Fresh and frozen vegetables have less added salt than canned vegetables. Drain and rinse canned vegetables if you want to remove some salt.
2. Choose more dark green and dark yellow vegetables, such as spinach, broccoli, romaine, carrots, chilies, and peppers.
3. Broccoli, brussels sprouts, cauliflower, greens, peppers, spinach, and tomatoes are good sources of vitamin C.
4. Vegetables contain 1 to 4 grams of fiber per serving.

Selection Tips

1. A 1-cup portion of broccoli is a portion about the size of a light bulb.
2. Tomato sauce is different from spaghetti sauce, which is on the Other Carbohydrates list.
3. Canned vegetables and juices are available without added salt.
4. If you eat 3 cups or more of raw vegetables or $1\frac{1}{2}$ cups of cooked vegetables at one meal, count them as 1 carbohydrate choice.
5. Starchy vegetables such as corn, peas, winter squash, and potatoes that contain larger amounts of calories and carbohydrates are on the Starch list.

One vegetable exchange equals
5 grams carbohydrate,
2 grams protein,
0 grams fat, and
25 calories.

Artichoke
Artichoke hearts
Asparagus
Beans (green, wax, Italian)
Bean sprouts
Beets
Broccoli
Brussels sprouts
Cabbage
Carrots
Cauliflower
Celery
Cucumber
Eggplant
Green onions or scallions
Greens (collard, kale, mustard, turnip)
Kohlrabi
Leeks
Mixed vegetables (without corn, peas, or pasta)

Mushrooms
Okra
Onions
Pea pods
Peppers (all varieties)
Radishes
Salad greens (endive, escarole, lettuce, romaine, spinach)
Sauerkraut★
Spinach
Summer squash
Tomato
Tomatoes, canned
Tomato sauce★
Tomato/vegetable juice★
Turnips
Water chestnuts
Watercress
Zucchini

★ = 400 mg or more sodium per exchange.

244

MEAT & MEAT SUBSTITUTES LIST

Meat and meat substitutes that contain both protein and fat are on this list. In general, one meat exchange is:
- 1 ounce meat, fish, poultry, or cheese,
- 1/2 cup beans, peas, and lentils.

Based on the amount of fat they contain, meats are divided into very lean, lean, medium-fat, and high-fat lists. This is done so you can see which ones contain the least amount of fat. One ounce (one exchange) of each of these includes:

	Carbohydrate (grams)	Protein (grams)	Fat (grams)	Calories
Very lean	0	7	0 to 1	35
Lean	0	7	3	55
Medium-fat	0	7	5	75
High-fat	0	7	8	100

Nutrition Tips

1. Choose very lean and lean meat choices whenever possible. Items from the high-fat group are high in saturated fat, cholesterol, and calories and can raise blood cholesterol levels.
2. Meats do not have any fiber.
3. Beans, peas, and lentils are good sources of fiber.
4. Some processed meats, seafood, and soy products may contain carbohydrate when consumed in large amounts. Check the Nutrition Facts on the label to see if the amount is close to 15 grams. If so, count it as a carbohydrate choice as well as a meat choice.

Selection Tips

1. Weigh meat after cooking and removing bones and fat. Four ounces of raw meat is equal to 3 ounces of cooked meat. Some examples of meat portions are:
   - 1 ounce cheese = 1 meat choice and is about the size of a 1-inch cube
   - 2 ounces meat = 2 meat choices, such as:
       1 small chicken leg or thigh
       1/2 cup cottage cheese or tuna
   - 3 ounces meat = 3 meat choices and is about the size of a deck of cards, such as:
       1 medium pork chop
       1 small hamburger
       1/2 of a whole chicken breast
       1 unbreaded fish fillet
2. Limit your choices from the high-fat group to three times per week or less.
3. Most grocery stores stock Select and Choice grades of meat. Select grades of meat are the leanest meats. Choice grades contain a moderate amount of fat, and Prime cuts of meat have the highest amount of fat. Restaurants usually serve Prime cuts of meat.
4. "Hamburger" may contain added seasoning and fat, but ground beef does not.
5. Read labels to find products that are low in fat and cholesterol (5 grams or less of fat per serving).
6. Beans, peas, and lentils are also found on the Starch list.

7. Peanut butter, in smaller amounts, is also found on the Fat list.
8. Bacon, in smaller amounts, is also found on the Fat list.

Meal Planning tips

1. Bake, roast, broil, grill, poach, steam, or boil these foods rather than frying.
2. Place meat on a rack so the fat will drain off during cooking.
3. Use a nonstick spray and a nonstick pan to brown or fry foods.
4. Trim off visible fat before or after cooking.
5. If you add flour, bread crumbs, coating mixes, fat or marinades when cooking, ask your dietitian how to count it in your meal plan.

Very Lean Meat & Substitutes List
One exchange equals 0 grams carbohydrate,
7 grams protein, 0 to 1 grams fat, & 35 calories.

**One very lean meat exchange is equal to
any one of the following items:**

Poultry: Chicken or turkey (white meat, no skin), Cornish hen (no skin)	1 ounce
Fish: Fresh or frozen cod, flounder, haddock, halibut, trout; tuna fresh or canned in water	1 ounce
Shellfish: Clams, crab, lobster, scallops, shrimp, imitation shellfish	1 ounce
Game: Duck or pheasant (no skin), venison, buffalo, ostrich	1 ounce
Cheese with 1 gram or less fat per ounce:	
Nonfat or low-fat cottage cheese	¼ cup
Fat-free cheese	1 ounce
Other: Processed sandwich meats with 1 gram or less fat per ounce, such as deli thin, shaved meats, chipped beef ♣, turkey ham	1 ounce
Egg whites	2
Egg substitutes, plain	¼ cup
Hot dogs with 1 gram or less fat per ounce ♣	1 ounce
Kidney (high in cholesterol)	1 ounce
Sausage with 1 gram or less fat per ounce	1 ounce

**Count as one very lean meat
and one starch exchange:**

Beans, peas, lentils (cooked)	½ cup

♣ = 400 mg or more sodium per exchange.

Lean Meat & Substitutes List
One exchange equals 0 grams carbohydrate,
7 grams protein, 3 grams fat, & 55 calories.

**One lean meat exchange is equal to
any one of the following items:**

Beef: USDA Select or Choice grades of lean beef (trimmed of fat), such as
round, sirloin, and flank steak; tenderloin; roast (rib, chuck, rump);
steak (T-bone, porterhouse, cubed), ground round   1 ounce
Pork: Lean pork, such as fresh ham; canned, cured, or boiled ham;
Canadian bacon♣; tenderloin, center loin chop   1 ounce
Lamb: Roast, chop, leg   1 ounce
Veal: Lean chop, roast   1 ounce
Poultry: Chicken, turkey (dark meat, no skin), chicken (white meat,
with skin), domestic duck or goose (well-drained of fat, no skin)   1 ounce
Fish: Herring (uncreamed or smoked)   1 ounce
    Oysters   6 medium
    Salmon (fresh or canned), catfish   1 ounce
    Sardines (canned)   2 medium
    Tuna (canned in oil, drained)   1 ounce
Game: Goose (no skin), rabbit   1 ounce
Cheese: 4.5%-fat cottage cheese $\frac{1}{4}$ cup
    Grated Parmesan   2 Tablespoons
    Cheeses with 3 grams or less fat per ounce   1 ounce
Other: Hot dogs with 3 grams or less fat per ounce ♣ $1\frac{1}{2}$ ounces
    Processed sandwich meat with 3 grams or less fat per ounce,
such as turkey pastrami or kielbasa   1 ounce
    Liver, heart (high in cholesterol)   1 ounce

♣ = 400 mg or more sodium per exchange.

Medium-Fat Meat & Substitutes List
One exchange equals 0 grams carbohydrate,
7 grams protein, 5 grams fat, & 75 calories.

**One medium-fat meat exchange is equal to
any one of the following items.**

Beef: Most beef products fall into this category (ground beef, meatloaf,
corned beef, short ribs, Prime grades of meat trimmed of fat,
such as prime rib)   1 ounce
Pork: Top loin, chop, Boston butt, cutlet   1 ounce
Lamb: Rib roast, ground   1 ounce
Veal: Cutlet (ground or cubed, unbreaded)   1 ounce
Poultry: Chicken (dark meat, with skin), ground turkey or
ground chicken, fried chicken (with skin)   1 ounce
Fish: Any fried fish product   1 ounce
Cheese: With 5 grams or less fat per ounce
    Feta   1 ounce
    Mozzarella   1 ounce
    Ricotta $\frac{1}{4}$ cup (2 ounces)

Other:

Egg (high in cholesterol, limit to 3 per week)	1
Sausage with 5 grams or less fat per ounce	1 ounce
Soy milk	1 cup
Tempeh	¼ cup
Tofu	4 ounces or ½ cup

High-Fat Meat & Substitutes List
One exchange equals 0 grams carbohydrate,
7 grams protein, 8 grams fat, & 100 calories.

Remember these items are high in saturated fat, cholesterol, and calories and may raise blood cholesterol levels if eaten on a regular basis.

**One high-fat meat exchange is equal to
any one of the following items.**

Pork: Spareribs, ground pork, pork sausage	1 ounce
Cheese: All regular cheeses, such as American✦,	
Cheddar, Monterey Jack, Swiss	1 ounce
Other: Processed sandwich meats with 8 grams or less fat per ounce	
such as bologna, pimento loaf, salami	1 ounce
Sausage, such as bratwurst, Italian, knockwurst, Polish, smoked	1 ounce
Hot dog (turkey or chicken)✦	1 (10/pound)
Bacon	3 slices (20 slices/pound)

**Count as one high-fat meat
plus one fat exchange.**

Hot dog (beef, pork, or combination)✦	1 (10/pound)
Peanut butter (contains unsaturated fat)	2 tablespoons

✦ = 400 mg or more sodium per exchange.

FAT LIST

Fats are divided into three groups, based on the main type of fat they contain: monounsaturated, polyunsaturated, and saturated. Small amounts of mono-unsaturated and polyunsaturated fats in the foods we eat are linked with good health benefits. Saturated fats are linked with heart disease and cancer. In general, one fat exchange is:

- 1 teaspoon of regular margarine or vegetable oil,
- 1 tablespoon of regular salad dressings.

Nutrition Tips
1. All fats are high in calories. Limit serving sizes for good nutrition and health.
2. Nuts and seeds contain small amounts of fiber, protein, and magnesium.
3. If blood pressure is a concern, choose fats in the unsalted form to help lower sodium intake, such as unsalted peanuts.

Selection Tips

1. Check the Nutrition Facts on food labels for serving sizes. One fat exchange is based on a serving size containing 5 grams of fat.
2. When selecting regular margarine, choose those with liquid vegetable table oil as the first ingredient. Soft margarines are not at saturated as stick margarine. Soft margarines are healthier choices. Avoid those listing hydrogenated partially hydrogenated fat as the first ingredient.
3. When selecting low-fat margarines, look for liquid vegetable oil as the second ingredient. Water is usually the first ingredient.
4. When used in smaller amounts, bacon and peanut butter are counted as fat choices. When used in larger amounts, they are counted as high-fat meat choices.
5. Fat-free salad dressings are on the Other Carbohydrates list and the Free Foods list.
6. See the Free Foods list for nondairy coffee creamers, whipped topping, and fat-free products, such as margarines, salad dressings, mayonnaise, sour cream, cream cheese, and nonstick cooking spray.

Monounsaturated, Polyunsaturated & Saturated Fats List
One fat exchange equals
5 grams fat & 45 calories.

MONOUNSATURATED FATS

Avocado (medium)	$1/8$ (1 ounce)
Oil (canola, olive, peanut)	1 teaspoon
Olives: ripe (black)	8 large
green (stuffed)♣	10 large
Nuts: almonds, cashews	6 nuts
mixed (50% peanuts)	6 nuts
peanuts	10 nuts
pecans	4 halves
Peanut butter (smooth or crunchy)	2 teaspoons
Sesame seeds	1 tablespoon
Tahini paste	2 teaspoons

POLYUNSATURATED FATS

Margarine: stick, tub, or squeeze	1 teaspoon
lower-fat (30% to 50% vegetable oil)	1 tablespoon
Mayonnaise (regular)	1 teaspoon
(reduced-fat)	1 tablespoon
Nuts (walnuts, English)	4 halves
Oil: corn, safflower, soybean	1 teaspoon
Salad dressing (regular)♣	1 tablespoon

(reduced-fat)	2 tablespoons
Miracle Whip Salad Dressing® (regular)	2 teaspoons
(reduced-fat)	1 tablespoon
Seeds: pumpkin, sunflower	1 tablespoon

♣ = 400 mg or more sodium per exchange.

SATURATED FATS LIST*

Bacon (cooked)	1 slice (20 slices/pound)
Bacon (grease)	1 teaspoon
Butter: stick	1 teaspoon
whipped	2 teaspoons
reduced-fat	1 tablespoon
Chitterlings (boiled)	2 tablespoons ($^1/_2$ ounce)
Coconut (sweetened, shredded)	2 tablespoons
Cream (half & half)	2 tablespoons
Cream cheese: regular	1 tablespoon ($^1/_2$ ounce)
reduced-fat	2 tablespoons (1 ounce)
Fatback or salt pork, see below†	
Shortening or lard	1 teaspoon
Sour cream: regular	2 tablespoons
reduced-fat	3 tablespoons

† Use a piece 1 inch x 1 inch X $^1/_4$ inch if you plan to eat the fatback cooked with vegetables. Use a piece 2 inches x 1 inch X $^1/_2$ inch when eating only the vegetables with the fatback removed.

*Saturated fats can raise blood cholesterol levels.

FREE FOODS LISTS

A *free food* is any food or drink that contains less than 20 calories or less than 5 grams of carbohydrate per serving. Foods with a serving size listed should be limited to three servings per day. Be sure to spread them out throughout the day. If you eat all three servings at one time, it could affect your blood glucose level. Foods listed without a serving size can be eaten as often as you like.

FAT-FREE OR REDUCED-FAT FOODS

Cream cheese (fat-free)	1 tablespoon
Creamers (nondairy, liquid)	1 tablespoon
Creamers (nondairy, powdered)	2 teaspoons
Mayonnaise: fat-free	1 tablespoon
reduced-fat	1 teaspoon
Margarine: fat-free	4 tablespoons
reduced-fat	1 teaspoon

Miracle Whip®: nonfat	1 tablespoon
reduced-fat	1 teaspoon
Nonstick cooking spray	
Salad dressing: fat-free	1 tablespoon
Italian (fat-free)	2 teaspoons
Salsa	¼ cup
Sour cream (fat-free, reduced-fat)	1 tablespoon
Whipped topping (regular or light)	2 tablespoons

SUGAR-FREE OR LOW-SUGAR FOODS

Candy (hard, sugar-free)	1 candy
Gelatin dessert (sugar-free)	
Gelatin (unflavored)	
Gum (sugar-free)	
Jam or jelly (low-sugar or light)	2 teaspoons
Sugar substitutes†	
Syrup (sugar-free)	2 tablespoons

†Sugar substitutes, alternatives, or replacements that are approved by the Food and Drug Administration (FDA) are safe to use. Common brand names include:

Equal® (aspartame)
Sprinkle Sweet® (saccharin)
Sweet One® (acesulfame K)
Sweet-10® (saccharin)
Sugar Twin® (saccharin)
Sweet 'n Low® (saccharin)

DRINKS

Bouillon (broth, consommé)⤵	
Bouillon or broth (low-sodium)	
Carbonated or mineral water	
Club soda	
Cocoa powder (unsweetened)	1 tablespoon
Coffee	
Diet soft drinks (sugar-free)	
Drink mixes (sugar-free)	
Tea	
Tonic water (sugar-free)	

CONDIMENTS

Catsup	1 tablespoon
Horseradish	
Lemon juice	
Lime juice	
Mustard	

EXCHANGE LISTS

Pickles (dill)♣   1½ large
Soy sauce (regular or light)♣
Taco sauce   1 tablespoon
Vinegar

SEASONINGS

Be careful with seasonings that contain sodium or are salts, such as garlic or celery salt, and lemon pepper.

Flavoring extracts
Garlic
Herbs (fresh or dried)
Pimento
Spices
Tabasco® or hot pepper sauce
Wine (used in cooking)
Worcestershire sauce

♣ = 400 mg or more of sodium per exchange.

INDEX